the little book of detox tips
for people on the go

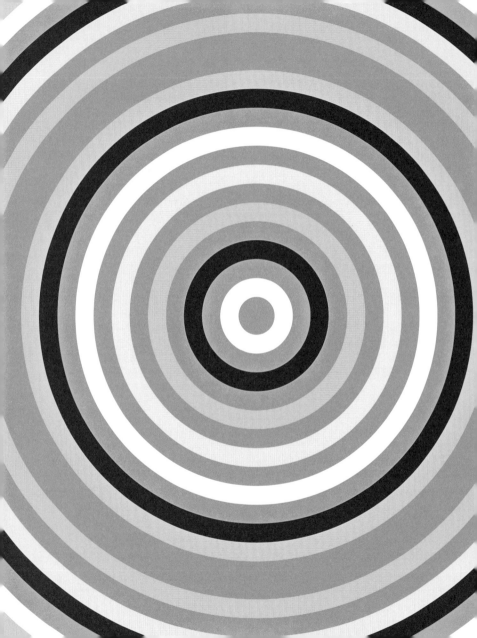

THE LITTLE BOOK OF
DETOX
TIPS

FOR PEOPLE ON THE GO

michael van
straten

quadrille

contents

introduction

There's nothing new about detoxing. The practice grew out of the ancient concept of fasting as the key to physical and spiritual cleansing – in other words, getting yourself squeaky-clean inside and out.

Detoxing is the modern take on fasting. A detox may start with a complete fast but not many people can spare a couple of weeks to devote to that type of total detox, which is why I have written this little book. It brings you a detox concept that's totally up to date, even if you can only spare a day or two.

Here I propose a completely safe but must shorter alternative to a total detox programme – in fact, there are three alternatives, depending on whether you want to make a difference to the status of your health, your energy levels or your radiance.

In addition you'll find a wealth of tips and hints for all the areas of your life that probably need attention if you can't always cope with 24/7 living.

There's advice – and recipes – so you eat what you should to get the most out of life and stay healthy, all the lowdown on supplements that give the extra boost we all need sometimes, and tips on how best to exercise, especially when you're short of time. You'll also find wellbeing pointers to ensure you get a good night's sleep and beat the stress, ideas for looking good – and not just by reaching for commercial lotions and potions – and lots of bite-size suggestions for coping with whatever home and work might throw at you.

Once you've had a go at my detox, you'll be hooked. Go on, give it a try.

Michael van Straten

detoxing

question why detox?

answer

If you suffer an occasional attack of the energy-droops – too many late nights, a few drinks too many, extra pressure at work, problems at home, the after-effects of a cold or of an attack of flu – you'll soon recover if you're healthy. But a detox will help you to get back on your feet. That's because fasting increases your natural resistance to infection, encourages the body to heal its damaged tissues and encourages homoeostasis – the mechanism that maintains the body's chemical stability, without which we couldn't survive.

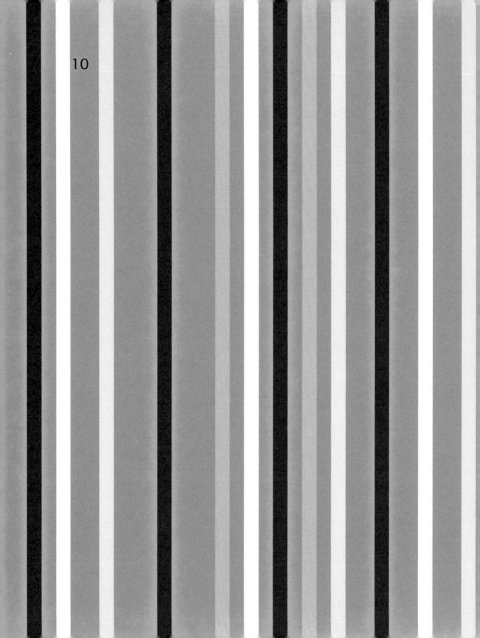

10

question when should I detox?

answer
A once-a-week 24-hour juice and water fast is the best way of maintaining good health. If that doesn't appeal to you, then a 48-hour regime, not more than once a month, is an extremely effective alternative. You can follow my 48-hour programme or you can just go for two days on water and juices, though by the end of the second day you'll feel a bit light-headed, so don't go in for any strenuous physical activity, drive or use dangerous machinery.

For a seasonal clear-out, a 3-day regime is ideal. Seek medical advice before starting if you've recently been ill. Don't do the 3-day fast while you're working and make sure to fit it in when you can have at least one day to recover. You could start at work on Friday, complete the fast on Saturday and Sunday, then have Monday as a day off.

extras while you detox

to maintain nutrient levels and increase energy

• Daily high-potency **multi-vitamin** and mineral supplement.

• **Co-enzyme Q** – a powerful antioxidant and especially valuable for chronic fatigue, glandular fever, tired-all-the-time syndrome and ME as it helps convert food into energy.

• **Guarana** – the extraordinary herb used as a source of energy by the Indians of the Brazilian rainforest for more than a thousand years. It's unique in its ability to produce gradual slow-release, long-term energy, rather than the quick boost and let-down that you get from a cup of strong coffee or a can of cola.

• **Ginseng** – used by the Chinese as an energy medicine for more than 6,000 years. It not only boosts physical and mental energy, but helps increase natural immunity and the body's ability to resist the damaging effects of stress.

for general wellbeing and improved elimination

• A one-a-day standardised extract of **cynarin** – from globe artichokes – to stimulate liver function and help the body eliminate fat-soluble substances stored in the liver.
• 1–2 tablespoons **oatbran** or **ground psyllium** or **flaxseed** every night while you detox. For best results, start the day before.
• **Parsley tea** (see page 17).

to boost immunity

• 500mg **vitamin C**, three times a day. If possible, take ester-C.
• **Echinacea** – one of the most effective herbs for short-term immunity boosting.
• **Probiotics** – beneficial bacteria that are key to strengthening your body's defence mechanisms.

14

rest and relaxation while you detox

Detoxing puts some strain on your physical resources, so it's essential to get enough rest while you're doing it. But there's a delicate balance to be struck. You need to be active to stimulate your heart, circulation and breathing, and get your liver working, but you mustn't overdo the physical exertion in the belief that you'll be detoxing more effectively. You won't. Your body will end up producing toxic chemical by-products, which will defeat the whole object.

Yes to – having a lie-in in the morning.

Yes to – putting your feet up for 10 minutes a few times a day.

Yes to – having a catnap during the day.

Yes to – going to bed a little earlier.

Yes to – two or three 10–15-minute walks a day.

No to – running or jogging.

No to – going to the gym.

No to – digging the garden.

No to – spring-cleaning the house.

No to – strenuous DIY.

drinking while you detox

You need to keep up your fluid intake while you're detoxing. Drink at least 1 1/2 litres water a day.

Yes to – filtered water, low-mineral-content bottled water or herb tea.

Yes to – Parsley Tea (see recipe opposite). Make up a jug first thing in the morning and drink small glasses regularly throughout the day to help speed up the detoxifying and cleansing processes. Make sure you drink it all.

No to – milk and sweeteners.

No to – canned drinks, squashes, fizzy water, cordials, Indian tea, coffee, and alcohol.

No to – sugar-free drinks since these contain artificial sweeteners.

parsley tea

Put 2 heaped tablespoons chopped fresh parsley in a large jug. Add 500ml boiling water, cover and leave to stand for 10 minutes. Strain, cool and keep covered in the fridge.

twenty-four hour cleansing for health

If you've had a week of entertaining clients, business lunches and over-indulgence, or you've been to a couple of great parties and had a bit too much alcohol, this 24-hour detox will flush out your system and revitalise your mind and body.

on waking A large glass of hot water with a thick slice of organic unwaxed lemon

breakfast A large glass of hot water with a thick slice of organic unwaxed lemon; a mug of Ginger Tea (see recipe opposite)

mid-morning A large glass of hot water with a thick slice of organic unwaxed lemon

lunch A large glass of Tomato Juice and Celery Blend (see recipe opposite); a mug of Ginger Tea (see recipe opposite)

mid-afternoon A large glass of hot water with a thick slice of organic unwaxed lemon

supper Kiwi and Pineapple Juice (see recipe opposite); a mug of Ginger Tea (see recipe opposite)

evening Orange Juice and Almond Blend (see recipe opposite)

bedtime A mug of any reputable brand of chamomile tea with a teaspoon of organic honey

ginger tea

Add 2.5cm fresh grated root ginger to a mug of boiling water. Cover and leave to stand for 5 minutes. Strain, add 1 tsp honey and sip slowly.

tomato juice and celery blend

6 large ripe plum tomatoes
2 stalks celery, with leaves
juice of 1 lemon
a dash of Tabasco (optional)

Simply put the tomatoes, celery and lemon juice in a blender or food processor and blend until smooth. Season to taste with the Tabasco sauce.

kiwi and pineapple juice

4 ripe kiwi fruit, peeled
1 pineapple, top removed

Cut the fruit into pieces and juice. Some heavy-duty juicers will cope with fruit with a tough skin like pineapples.

orange juice and almond blend

4 large oranges, juiced
4 tbsp ground almonds

Simply mix the two ingredients together and whisk with a fork.

forty-eight hour cleansing **for health**

If a one-day-a-week detox doesn't appeal to you, you might prefer a 48-hour regime that you do once a month. Start by following the 24-Hour Cleansing for Health regime. **On Day 2 have:**

on waking A large glass of hot water with a thick slice of organic unwaxed lemon

breakfast A large glass of hot water with a thick slice of organic unwaxed lemon; an orange; half a pink grapefruit; a slice of cantaloupe melon; a mug of chamomile tea

mid-morning A large glass of hot water with a thick slice of organic unwaxed lemon

lunch A large plate of mixed raw red and yellow pepper, cucumber, carrot, radishes, tomatoes, celery and broccoli, with a handful of chopped fresh parsley and a drizzle of extra-virgin olive oil and lemon juice; a large glass of apple juice; a mug of mint tea

mid-afternoon A large glass of hot water with a thick slice of organic unwaxed lemon

supper A large bowl of fresh fruit salad, to include apple, pear, grapes, mango and some berries – but no banana; a handful of raisins – make sure to chew them very slowly – and a handful of fresh, unsalted cashew nuts; a glass of unsalted mixed vegetable juice (any reputable brand)

evening A large glass of hot water with a thick slice of organic unwaxed lemon

bedtime A mug of any reputable brand of chamomile tea with a teaspoon of organic honey

three-day cleansing
for health

Start by following the 48-Hour Cleansing for Health programme on pages 20–21. **On day 3:**

on waking A large glass of hot water with a thick slice of organic unwaxed lemon

breakfast A large glass of hot water with a thick slice of organic unwaxed lemon; a carton of organic low-fat live yoghurt with a teaspoon of honey, a dessertspoon of raisins and a dessertspoon of chopped hazelnuts; a glass of half-orange, half-grapefruit juice

mid-morning A large glass of Carrot, Apple and Celery Juice (see recipe page 25); 4 dried apricots; 4 prunes

lunch A large glass of hot water with a slice of organic unwaxed lemon; Carrot and Red Cabbage Salad (see recipe page 25); a mug of mint tea

mid-afternoon A glass of any unsweetened fruit juice

supper A mixture of chopped steamed leek, cabbage, spinach and kale, drizzled with olive oil, lemon juice and a generous sprinkling of nutmeg; a glass of unsweetened red grape juice; a mug of lime-blossom tea

evening 4 prunes; 4 dates; a small bunch of black grapes

bedtime A cup of China tea with two rice crackers

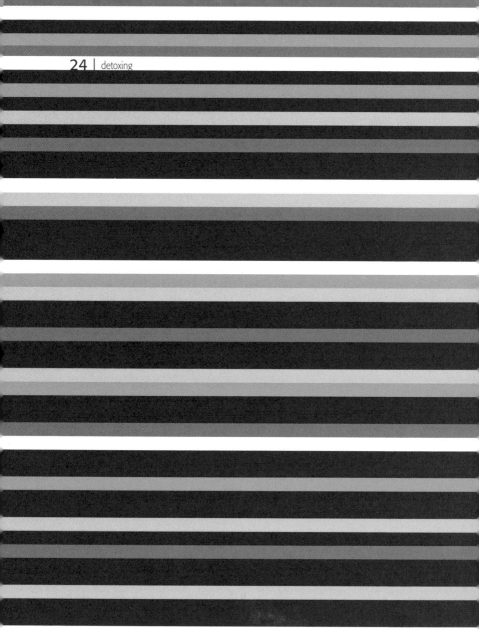

carrot and red cabbage salad

2 large carrots, grated
1/2 red cabbage, finely
  shredded
2 apples, peeled and
  finely grated
1 red pepper, deseeded
  and finely cubed
4 plum tomatoes,
  quartered
10 radishes, quartered
2 celery stalks, finely
  chopped
2 tbsp sunflower seeds
6 tbsp extra-virgin
  olive oil
juice of 1/2 lemon

Mix the first 7 ingredients together in a bowl and blend thoroughly. Sprinkle the sunflower seeds on top. Whisk the olive oil and lemon juice together in a separate bowl, drizzle over the salad and serve.

carrot, apple and celery juice

3 large carrots, topped
  and tailed – and
  peeled if not organic
2 apples, quartered
2 celery stalks

Put all the ingredients in a blender or liquidiser and whizz together until smooth.

twenty-four hour cleansing for energy

The day before your 24-Hour Cleansing for Energy detox, avoid all animal protein and have a fairly light diet of just fruit, vegetables and salads.

on waking A large glass of hot water with a thick slice of organic unwaxed lemon

breakfast A large glass of hot water with a thick slice of organic unwaxed lemon; a glass of unsweetened pineapple juice

mid-morning A large glass of hot water with a thick slice of organic unwaxed lemon

lunch A large glass of hot water with a thick slice of organic unwaxed lemon; a large glass of any salt-free vegetable juice; a mug of ginseng tea

mid-afternoon A large glass of hot water with a thick slice of organic unwaxed lemon

supper Mango, Kiwi and Pineapple Juice (see recipe opposite); a mug of any reputable brand of raspberry leaf tea

evening A large glass of hot water with a thick slice of organic unwaxed lemon; Carrot, Apple and Celery Juice (see recipe page 25)

bedtime A mug of any reputable brand of chamomile tea

mango, kiwi and pineapple juice

1 large ripe mango,
stoned
4 kiwi fruit, peeled
1 medium pineapple,
top removed

Simply put all the
ingredients in a blender
or liquidiser and whizz
together until smooth.

forty-eight hour cleansing for energy

Start by following the 24-Hour Cleansing for Energy regime. **On day 2 have:**

on waking A large glass of hot water with a thick slice of organic unwaxed lemon

breakfast A large glass of hot water with a thick slice of organic unwaxed lemon and quarter of a teaspoon of powdered cinnamon – this tends to float on top of the water even if you stir; a large bunch of grapes; a mug of lemon and ginger tea

mid-morning A large glass of hot water with a thick slice of organic unwaxed lemon

lunch An apple, a stick of celery and 6 radishes; a large glass of tomato juice; a mug of mint tea

mid-afternoon A large glass of hot water with a thick slice of organic unwaxed lemon

supper A mango, 60g blueberries and a pear; 4 ready-to-eat prunes; a glass of unsalted mixed vegetable juice

evening A large glass of hot water with a thick slice of organic unwaxed lemon; Hauser Broth (see recipe opposite)

bedtime A mug of any reputable brand of chamomile tea with a teaspoon of organic honey

hauser broth

Gaylord Hauser was one of the pioneering American naturopaths during the golden era of Hollywood. All the great stars of the 1940s, 1950s and 1960s flocked to see him. He gave me this recipe, which he used in his fasting regimes as an energy booster.

125g carrots
3 stalks celery, finely chopped with leaves
75g spinach or chard leaves, finely chopped
1.5 litres water
1 level tbsp runny honey
2 tbsp tomato purée
1 tbsp chives, finely snipped

Put the carrots, celery and spinach or chard into a saucepan with the water. Simmer for 30 minutes. Add the tomato purée and honey and cook for a further 5 minutes. Transfer the soup to a blender or food processor and whizz until smooth. Ladle into soup bowls, sprinkle the snipped chives on top and serve.

three-day cleansing
for energy

When it comes to boosting your energy levels, it really does pay to go straight into the 3-day Cleansing for Energy detox plan if at all possible. When you wake up on the morning of day 4, you'll feel like a new person. Be careful though. The temptation to do all those things you've been putting off for months must be resisted, otherwise you'll dissipate all the benefits that you've worked so hard for. Take things gently and ease yourself gradually back into your normal routine.

Start by following the 48-Hour Cleansing for Energy regime.
On Day 3 have:

on waking A large glass of hot water with a thick slice of organic unwaxed lemon

breakfast A large glass of hot water with a thick slice of organic unwaxed lemon; half a cantaloupe melon filled with fresh berries; a mug of rosehip tea

mid-morning Carrot, Apple and Beetroot Juice (see recipe page 32)

lunch A large glass of hot water with a thick slice of organic unwaxed lemon; a bowl of Porridge with Cinnamon and Dried Fruits made with water (see recipe page 33); a large glass of tomato juice

mid-afternoon A large glass of hot water with a thick slice of organic unwaxed lemon

supper A large glass of hot water with a thick slice of organic unwaxed lemon; a mixture of chopped steamed leek, cabbage, spinach and kale, drizzled with olive oil and lemon juice and with a generous sprinkling of nutmeg; a large glass of carrot juice; a mug of mint tea

evening 4 each dried or soaked prunes and apricots

bedtime 1 slice of wholemeal bread with a little honey; a mug of mint tea

carrot, apple and beetroot juice

It's the high natural sugar content of the beetroot that makes this juice an energy booster. But there's an added bonus in the form of the skin-friendly vitamin A in the carrots.

3 large carrots, topped and tailed, and peeled if not organic
2 apples, quartered
2 small beetroot, raw with leaves

Simply put all the ingredients in a blender or liquidiser and whizz together until smooth.

porridge with cinnamon and dried fruits

This has all the energy and blood sugar benefits of the oats, plus the huge antioxidant and protective value of the fruits.

2 average cups
    porridge oats
2 average cups semi-
    skimmed milk
2 average cups water
150g mixed dried fruits
2 level tsp ground
    cinnamon

Put the oats, milk and water into a saucepan. Bring to the boil and simmer for 5 minutes or according to the packet instructions, stirring regularly. While it's cooking, cut the dried fruits into evenly sized pieces, about as big as a little fingernail. When the porridge is cooked, stir in the fruit and 1 tsp cinnamon. Cover and leave to rest for 2 minutes. Serve with the remaining cinnamon sprinkled on top and extra milk, if desired.

twenty-four hour cleansing for radiance

Whether you use this 24-Hour Cleansing for Radiance fast as a regular radiance boost or feel you need it because you've just had a weekend of rich food and too much alcohol, you'll find it's really worth the effort – just take a look in the mirror 24 hours later to see the difference.

on waking A large glass of hot water with a thick slice of organic unwaxed lemon

breakfast A large glass of hot water with a thick slice of organic unwaxed lemon; a glass of Radiant Juice (see recipe opposite); a mug of nettle tea

mid-morning A large glass of hot water with a thick slice of organic unwaxed lemon

lunch A large glass of Tomato Juice with Garlic and Spring Onions (see recipe opposite); a mug of nettle tea

mid-afternoon A large glass of hot water with a thick slice of organic unwaxed lemon

supper Mango, Kiwi and Pineapple Juice (see recipe page 27); a mug of nettle tea

evening Carrot and Beetroot Juice (see recipe opposite)

bedtime A mug of lime-blossom tea

radiant juice

1 large dessert apple,
  quartered
1 orange, peeled but
  with some pith
2 large carrots, topped,
  tailed and peeled if
  not organic
2.5cm fresh root ginger,
  peeled and sliced

Put the ingredients into a
blender or liquidiser and
whizz until smooth.

tomato juice with garlic and spring onions

8 large tomatoes
2 fat bulbs spring
  onions, trimmed
4 large sprigs basil
6 large sprigs oregano

Roughly chop the tomatoes
and spring onions and put
into a blender or liquidiser
with the leaves from the
basil and oregano. Whizz
until smooth.

carrot and beetroot juice

4 carrots, topped and
  tailed
4 medium beetroot
3 large sprigs basil

Put the ingredients into a
blender or liquidiser and
whizz until smooth.

forty-eight hour cleansing
for radiance

Start by following the 24-Hour Cleansing for Radiance regime.
On Day 2 have:

on waking A large glass of hot water with a thick slice of organic unwaxed lemon

breakfast A large glass of hot water with a thick slice of organic unwaxed lemon; a large glass of Radiant Juice (see recipe page 35); a mug of nettle tea

mid-morning A large glass of hot water with a thick slice of organic unwaxed lemon

lunch A glass of Radiant Lemonade (see recipe opposite); a mug of mint tea

mid-afternoon A large glass of hot water with a thick slice of organic unwaxed lemon

supper A large bowl of fresh fruit salad, to include apple, pear, grapes, mango and some berries – but no banana; a handful of raisins – chew them very slowly – and a handful of fresh, unsalted cashew nuts; a mug of mint tea

evening A large glass of hot water with a thick slice of organic unwaxed lemon

bedtime A mug of any reputable brand of chamomile tea with a teaspoon of organic honey

radiant lemonade

Vitamin A is essential for healthy, radiant skin and you'll get it in abundance from the carrots in this juice. The bonus comes from the radishes – their natural constituents stimulate the cleansing function of the liver, making this the perfect juice when you've been a bit over-indulgent or your digestive system seems slightly sluggish.

1 large carrot, topped, tailed and peeled if not organic
10 radishes, topped and tailed
1 apple, quartered
1 beetroot, topped and tailed
juice and finely grated zest of 2 lemons
up to 300ml naturally sparkling mineral water (optional)

Juice the first 4 ingredients. Add the lemon juice and zest. If you want a longer, fizzy drink, add the mineral water.

three-day cleansing
for radiance

When you wake up on day four after this cleansing regime, your body will feel lighter, your system cleaner and your eyes and skin will have a sparkle and lustre you haven't seen in ages. You'll also be overflowing with all the protective antioxidants you need and you'll almost certainly have lost more than a kilo in weight.

Start by following the 48-Hour Cleansing for Radiance regime. **On Day 3 have:**

on waking A large glass of hot water with a thick slice of organic unwaxed lemon

breakfast A large glass of hot water with a thick slice of organic unwaxed lemon; fresh fruit salad – a mixture of any of the following: apple, pear, grapes, mango and pineapple and any berries, with a carton of live yoghurt and a tablespoon of unsweetened muesli; a cup of weak Indian tea or herb tea

mid-morning 6 dried apricots; a glass of fruit or vegetable juice

lunch Watercress Soup (see recipe, page 40) with a chunk of crusty wholemeal bread, no butter; a cup of weak Indian tea or herb tea

mid-afternoon An apple and a pear

supper Courgette Pasta (see recipe, page 41); a salad of tomato, onion and yellow pepper; a cup of weak Indian tea or herb tea

watercress soup

Watercress is one of the truly great radiant foods. It's hugely antioxidant, especially protective against lung cancer, and rich in iron, which makes it a key to inner beauty.

1 tbsp olive oil
1 medium onion, finely chopped
2 cloves garlic, finely chopped
3 bunches watercress, with stalks
1 litre vegetable stock
200g live natural yoghurt

Heat the oil in a large saucepan and sauté the onion gently until soft. Add the garlic and continue to cook for 2 minutes. Add the watercress and continue to cook gently until it wilts. Add the stock and simmer for about 10 minutes. Transfer to a blender or food processor and whizz until smooth. Serve hot or cold with a swirl of yoghurt in each bowl.

courgette pasta

400g thin pasta, such
   as spaghettini
4 medium courgettes,
   grated
3cm fresh root ginger,
   grated
4 tsp extra-virgin
   olive oil
4 tsp Parmesan cheese,
   freshly grated
4 spring onions, finely
   chopped
125g beansprouts

Cook the pasta in a saucepan of boiling water according to the packet instructions. Transfer to a large serving bowl and mix in all the other ingredients. Serve immediately.

42

the 12 rules for replenishing

1 After you have detoxed, you need to spend the next seven days replenishing your body.

2 You don't have to follow a rigid regime but you must eat breakfast, one light meal and one main meal a day.

3 You should eat small amounts at a time, but often.

4 You should avoid eating the same foods every day to ensure that you have as wide a spread as possible of essential vitamins, minerals and trace elements.

5 You should drink 1.5 litres a day, of which 1 litre must be water. You can now drink a total of 5 cups of real tea and coffee, but not more than 3 of coffee.

6 You may have some alcohol, but no more than 21 units a week if you're a man, and no more than 14 units a week if you're a woman.

7 Finish every meal with a generous portion of fresh or cooked fruit.

8 At least 700g of what you eat each day should consist of fruit, vegetables and salad.

9 Half your calories should come from complex carbohydrates – bread, pasta, rice, beans and so on.

10 If you are a vegetarian, don't overdo the eggs and the cheese and if you're a carnivore, eat meat, fish and poultry, but in modest amounts.

11 During this week, avoid the 'anti-nutrients' – the foods such as takeaways, burgers, fries, crisps, high-sugar cakes, biscuits and pastries. All of these sap your health and vitality.

12 Eat as little ready-made convenience food as possible.

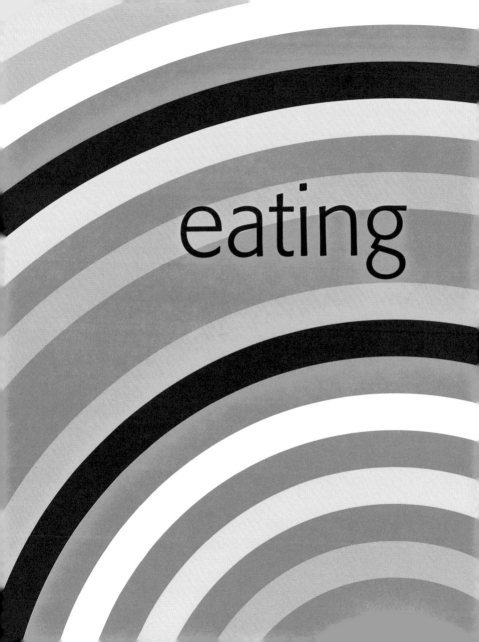

eating

the three-box trick

Next time you go shopping, try the three-box trick for family food shopping. Put three equal-sized boxes in your supermarket trolley.

Box 1 Fill to the brim with good-quality carbohydrates – potatoes, rice, pasta, bread, beans, and good cereals such as porridge, muesli, wholegrain breakfast cereals and wholewheat flakes.

Box 2 This must overflow with fruit, vegetables and salads. You should also include dried fruits, fresh nuts and seeds. Frozen vegetables are fine as they are almost as nutritious as fresh.

Box 3 Imagine this box is divided into three compartments – two compartments each take up 40 per cent of the space and the third takes up the last 20 per cent. Put your cheese, milk, yoghurt and eggs in the first of the large compartments and your meat, fish and poultry or vegetarian protein – tofu, Quorn™ or textured vegetable protein (TVP) in the second. Cream, biscuits, sweets, chocolates, sticky buns and other treats go in the last small compartment.

Use the same proportions for your daily diet. That way you'll get at least half your calories from good carbohydrates, no more than a third of them from fat, and between 10 and 12 per cent of them from protein. Add a couple of glasses of wine a day and your calories from alcohol will be less than 10 per cent of your daily calorie intake and won't exceed the recommended maximum number of units.

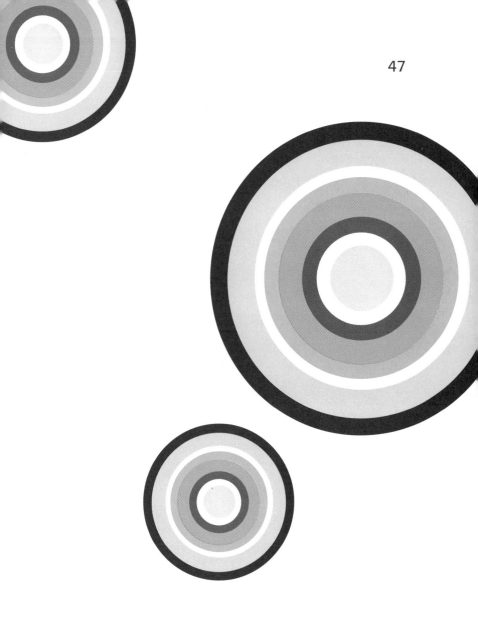

did you know that…?

….today, many of us are overfed yet undernourished. In the days of our great-grandparents and grandparents, there was less obesity, less heart disease, less cancer – and eating disorders were virtually unknown. People only ate food that was in season and mothers relied on their common sense and on the skills they'd learned from their mothers to raise healthy, well-fed families.

down with extremism

American paediatricians are already dealing with parents they label 'chemophobes' – people who are so obsessive about only giving their children organic food that if they can't find organic fruit and vegetables, they would rather give them none at all. This is madness: the risks of depriving children of fresh produce are far greater than any risks caused by chemical residues.

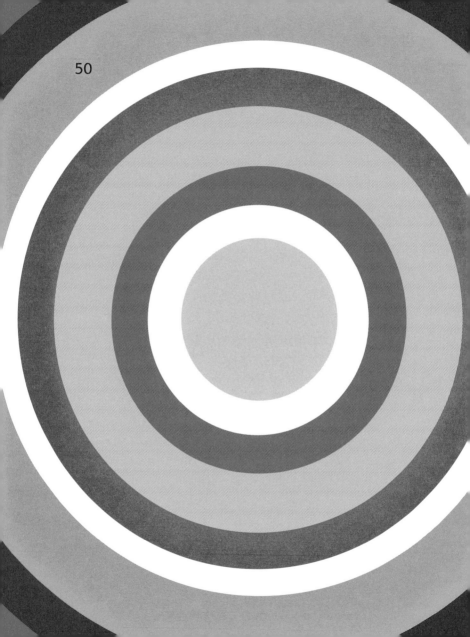

50

eight top herbs for health – and one spice for luck!

1 Sage improves the digestion of fats.

2 Mint is a powerful antacid and prevents indigestion.

3 Basil calms you down and makes you feel good.

4 Bay leaves are helpful for chest infections.

5 Garlic lowers cholesterol.

6 Coriander is good for wind and is reputedly an aphrodisiac.

7 Dill is great for irritable bowel syndrome.

8 Parsley is a diuretic and helps with premenstrual puffiness.

– and **ginger** is the perfect cure for early morning sickness during pregnancy or travel sickness.

question are carbohydrates really bad for me?

answer Bread, potatoes, rice, pasta and cereals are not fattening or unhealthy. It's what you do to them that makes the difference. Potatoes drizzled with olive oil, sprinkled with rosemary and roasted in the oven are wonderful. Pasta with sauce made from tomatoes, vegetables or fish is great food. Good wholemeal bread with a thin smear of butter is delicious and highly nutritious. Just don't overdo the portion size and go easy on the oil and butter.

question are convenience foods really bad for me?

answer You shouldn't rely exclusively on ready-made meals, takeaways or convenience foods. Some convenience foods though are better than others and should always be in your kitchen cupboard, for instance canned tomatoes, canned fish of all sorts and canned beans, like baked beans, kidney beans, borlotti beans and chickpeas (rinse well to remove the salt). With these convenience foods around, if you always have some spring onions, garlic, cucumber, a pepper and your favourite salad dressing handy, it's easy to rustle up a healthy nourishing instant meal.

question is salt really bad for me?

answer Watch the labels for salt content. Salt is known to be a major factor in causing high blood pressure and strokes, so aim for 4g a day maximum (the average intake in Western countries is 12g). Once you start looking, you'll be amazed where salt crops up. Some brands of cornflakes, for example, have more salt in one bowl than the equivalent amount of seawater. So throw away the salt cellar and enjoy the wonderful flavours of the food itself, enhanced just by spices and fresh herbs.

question what are good calories?

answer

The healthiest calories come from complex carbohydrates like wholemeal bread, oats, potatoes, pasta, rice and beans. They should make up at least half your daily food, but there is a limit to how much you can eat at one time. Get extra calories from bananas, unsalted nuts and dried fruits. Raisins, sultanas, dates and dried apricots are excellent sources of vitamins, minerals and fibre and, eaten as snacks and nibbles, they add a significant number of calories in a comparatively small amount of food.

Other sources of healthy calories are seeds. Sunflower and sesame seeds are especially good, and peanut butter and tahini – a spread made from crushed sesame – provide a large number of calories, plenty of essential rebuilding nutrients and very little bulk.

question why are so many people overweight?

answer Although many of us now consume 800 calories a day less than people did in the 1950s, we're eating 50 per cent more fat, and almost all of us, including children, are far less physically active, both at work and leisure. And while the slimming industry pushes the 'lose-weight' messages, the multinational food industry encourages an ever-increasing consumption of high-fat, high-sugar convenience and junk foods.

three sure-fire weight-loss tips

1 If you eat two slices of bread and butter a day less and walk 15 minutes a day more, you'll lose half a kilo a week without doing anything else.

2 If you stand up whenever you speak on the telephone, you'll lose over two kilos a year. It takes more muscle effort to stand than sit!

3 And if you use a remote control for your TV, you'll gain a kilo a year – so throw the remote away.

yo-yo dieting

There are no miracle diets, though it's true that there are some that make you lose weight quickly. Unfortunately, they're either unhealthy, unsustainable or both, and the minute you stop dieting, you put back on all the weight you've lost, plus a kilo or two. And each time you do that, your fat deposits move further up your body, so you gradually change from a healthy pear shape to an unhealthy apple shape – the more fat you carry around your middle, the greater the risk of heart disease. You have been warned!

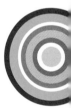

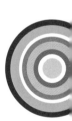

the only thing you have to do to get the weight off – and keep it off

Forget the cabbage-soup diet – it's antisocial. Forget high-protein diets – they can seriously damage your kidneys. And forget eating for your blood group, eating nothing but fruit before lunch and any other cranky diet idea that flies in the face of normal balanced eating. All you have to do to keep your weight under control is to eat good, healthy food on a regular basis.

question am I allowed the occasional lapse
when I'm trying to lose weight?

answer

Of course you are. Just remember, it's what you
eat most of the time that counts – what you eat
occasionally doesn't matter a damn.

question how can I gain weight?

answer Be a grazer. Aim to eat something at least every two hours, starting with a really good breakfast and finishing with a bedtime snack. Dips like guacamole, made from avocado and olive oil, or hummus, made with chickpeas and tahini, eaten with wholemeal pitta bread, make excellent between-meals snacks and, like all the best foods, provide a high proportion of nutrients together with their calories.

drink this

If you suffer severe embarrassment through being underweight, here's my healthy weight-gain secret weapon. It's also excellent for anyone undergoing chemotherapy who may not feel like or be able to eat 'proper' food. Make it up first thing in the morning, drink a glass of it before breakfast, keep the rest in the fridge and make sure it's all gone by bedtime.

$^1/_2$ litre whole milk
1 certified salmonella-free raw egg
1 banana
1 dessertspoon molasses
1 dessertspoon honey
1 dessertspoon tahini
1 dessertspoon wheatgerm
1 dessertspoon brewer's yeast powder
4 dried apricots

Whizz all the ingredients together in a blender and enjoy.

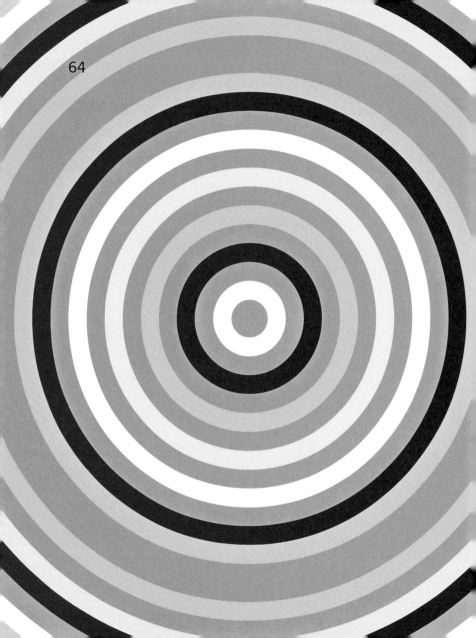

64

six reasons why you should always eat breakfast

1 When you get up in the morning, it may be 8–12 hours since you last ate and your blood-sugar level is at rock bottom. For your brain to function properly it needs a constant supply of sugar, which is why starting your day with breakfast is so important.

2 While you sleep, your body is working hard as this is the time for growth and repair. Your brain switches off the activity hormones and turns on to maintenance mode. While all this work is going on, you are using up your reserves of vital nutrients, so your storehouse needs replenishing, which is why breakfast is the most important meal of the day.

3 Skipping breakfast means poorer performance by schoolchildren.

4 Skipping breakfast means a greater risk of accidents when driving.

5 Skipping breakfast means a lack of efficiency at work.

6 Skipping breakfast means irritability.

scary statistics

- **5,000,000** – the number of people who don't bother to eat breakfast but grab a snack while dashing to work

- **1,500,000** – the number of bacon sandwiches consumed each day for breakfast in the UK

- **1,000,000 +** – the number of packets of crisps consumed each day for breakfast in the UK

- **1,000,000 +** – the number of sugary soft drinks consumed each day for breakfast in the UK

- **500,000** – the number of bags of sweets or bars of chocolate consumed each day for breakfast in the UK

- **50 %** – the percentage of people at work in the UK who don't eat anything for breakfast

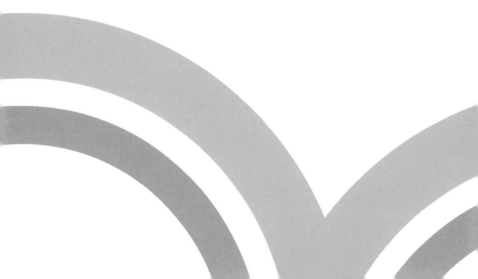

overnight muesli

The slow-release energy from the oats makes them perfect for breakfast or brunch as they help keep your blood sugar on an even keel for several hours. This means you avoid those mid-morning sugar cravings.

12 heaped tbsp organic, low-salt, unsweetened muesli
about 500ml apple juice
about 500g live natural yoghurt

Put the muesli into 2 bowls. Pour on the apple juice – don't worry if the mixture seems very runny; the cereal will expand. Stir in the yoghurt and leave in the fridge overnight.

did you know that...?

....what you eat for breakfast can influence the way you perform during the day?

Replenishing your protein means real energy and brain activity, whereas a mainly starch-based breakfast keeps you calm, serene and happy.

the sporting breakfast

If you take your exercise early in the day, the essential ingredient in your breakfast should be lots of healthy calories and a fairly modest amount of protein, so the ideal start for you is a large bowl of porridge or muesli with 3 prunes, 3 dried apricots, a handful of sultanas or raisins and a generous sprinkling of mixed sunflower and pumpkin seeds for extra minerals. Follow with a matchbox-sized piece of cheese and an apple, and take a banana with you to replace the energy and potassium after your exercise.

the expectant breakfast

During pregnancy you need extra energy as well as extra nutrients. A small pot of plain live yoghurt with a generous dessertspoon of runny honey drizzled on the top and a sprinkling of mixed chopped, unsalted, unroasted fresh nuts will get you off to a good start. This will provide energy, protein, calcium, vitamin E and lots of other essential nutrients. Follow with at least one thick slice of good wholemeal or rye toast spread with organic peanut butter – yes, it's extremely healthy and a great source of instant energy – and a glass of fresh unsweetened fruit juice or unsalted vegetable juice.

the power breakfast

If you start your working day by going straight into a high-powered meeting that requires your brain to be bursting with energy, you need a high-protein breakfast, but avoid the traditional high-fat, high-cholesterol, artery-clogging frying-pan breakfast, and skip the waffles and cream. Poached eggs, griddled bacon, a grilled low-fat sausage with grilled tomatoes and mushrooms, a glass of juice, and two slices of good wholemeal toast will get you off to a flying start. The protein will stimulate your brain activity and energetic thought and you'll be unstoppable!

question what's this thing called glucose?

answer

Glucose – or blood sugar as it is also confusingly known – is the fuel our bodies run on. The glucose circulating in our bloodstream after a carbohydrate meal is circulated to cells for instant use, and any surplus is converted into glycogen and stored as fuel in the liver, ready to be 'switched on' whenever it is needed. The hormone insulin, secreted by the pancreas, is responsible for this storage job.

question what's this thing called hypoglycaemia?

answer Have you ever tucked into a couple of biscuits, a bowl of cornflakes or a chocolate bar? I bet you have. If so, you may have noticed how, a little later, you're full of pep and a few hours after that, you're jittery and dying for a little sugary fix. That's because you're now suffering – if only in passing – from hypoglycaemia or low blood-sugar, sometimes called the 'Sugar Blues'.

When you eat carbohydrates, the sugars they contain are broken down into glucose during digestion. Eat a slice of wholegrain bread, a dish of lentils or a handful of ripe apricots, and their sugars are broken down into glucose quite slowly. But when you eat your biscuits, cornflakes or chocolate – the high-glycaemic foods – their sugars are broken down very quickly, sending the glucose levels in your bloodstream rocketing. The pancreas then pumps out extra insulin to help it cope and your blood-sugar levels drop sharply – giving you the 'Sugar Blues'.

question why should I care about my blood-sugar level?

answer Fluctuations in blood-sugar levels caused by eating high-glycaemic foods (see page 73) have been linked with a huge spectrum of health problems. Long-term, they can be responsible for high blood pressure, obesity, diabetes and heart disease. In children they may be responsible for disruptive behaviour, hyperactivity and an inability to concentrate. And one of the commonest symptoms of low blood sugar is mental and physical fatigue – which may account for the state of permanent exhaustion suffered by so many adults, teenagers and children.

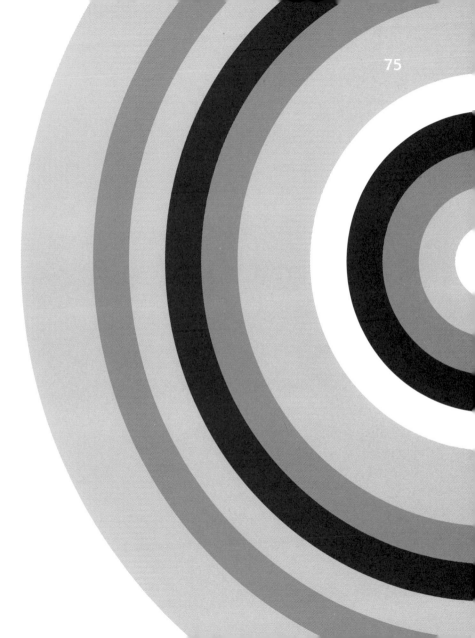

idiot's guide to the glycaemic index

• The glycaemic index – GI – is a way of calculating the rate at which carbohydrates are digested and converted into sugar by the body.

• The lower a food's GI, the longer it takes for that food to be converted into sugar.

• Taking 100 as the standard, processed foods like white bread, sugared breakfast cereals, puffed rice, cornflakes, puffed wheat, sweet biscuits, instant mashed potato, corn chips, glucose and honey, all have a GI between 70 and 100.

• Foods with a GI below 60 are wholemeal wheat, rye and pumpernickel, wholemeal pasta, brown rice, sweetcorn, buckwheat, bulgur, wholewheat kernels, whole rye kernels, pearl barley, shredded wheat, oatmeal, chickpeas, soya beans, all dried beans, and low-fat dairy foods.

• By mixing low GI foods into a meal, you'll be able to maintain a much more even level of blood sugar and so ensure a constant flow of mental and physical energy.

pasta all'aglio e olio

This recipe is just as good for your health as it is for boosting your energy, which it will do for two to three hours. The health-giving fats in the olive oil take even longer to convert to useable energy, so you get an extra spurt just when you've used up the energy provided by the pasta.

400g spaghettini
6 tbsp extra-virgin olive oil
3 cloves garlic, peeled and crushed with the flat blade of a broad knife
4 tbsp freshly grated Parmesan cheese
6 large sprigs basil, leaves removed and finely torn

Cook the pasta according to the packet instructions. Meanwhile, heat the olive oil in a saucepan, add the garlic and cook gently until just beginning to turn brown. Remove the garlic with a slotted spoon and discard. Pour the hot oil over the pasta and mix thoroughly. Stir in the Parmesan cheese and mix again. Finally, stir in the basil leaves and serve immediately.

squash, almond and raisin bulgur

This energy-giving vegetable dish is another
fast/slow energy meal – thanks to the fruit, the
sugar and the grains. If you've never cooked
with bulgur before, do try this recipe. Bulgur is
a wonderful wheat, and cooking it is as easy
as cooking rice.

150g bulgur
at least 6 tbsp olive oil
2 large, very finely
    sliced onions
350g peeled, deseeded
    and cubed squash or
    courgettes
12 tsp ground
    coriander
12 tsp ground cumin
150g flaked almonds
110g raisins
salt and black pepper

Simmer the bulgur in twice
its volume of water for 10
minutes. Heat 2 tbsp of the
oil and fry the onion until
brown. Add the squash and
sauté until brown, adding
more oil if necessary. Add
the spices and cook for 1
minute, stirring all the time.
Reduce the heat, add the
almonds and raisins and
cook, still stirring, until the
almonds are golden. Drain
the bulgur, if necessary. Stir
into the vegetables. Season
to taste with salt and black
pepper. Add more oil if the
mixture looks too dry and
heat through for 1 minute.

four white flour facts…

Foods such as wholegrain bread, brown rice, whole oats, beans and lentils and fruits are loaded with important nutrients and are rich in fibre, which helps keep the digestive system functioning efficiently. But when these foods are refined or heavily processed, which is what happens when white flour is made, they lose not only a whole slew of vital nutrients, but most of the fibre too.

1 White flour contains much less zinc than wholemeal flour. Zinc is essential for resistance, mental energy and male sexual function.

2 White flour contains much less magnesium than wholemeal flour. Magnesium is vital for the nervous system and also for the absorption of calcium

3 White flour contains significantly less protein than wholemeal flour. Protein is essential for body-building.

4 Token amounts of major nutrients are added back when white flour is baked into bread, but not when it goes into other foods.

…and all you need to know about white sugar

White sugar has absolutely no nutritional value at all. It's just full of 'empty' calories. Brown sugar and honey at least contain traces of some key nutrients.

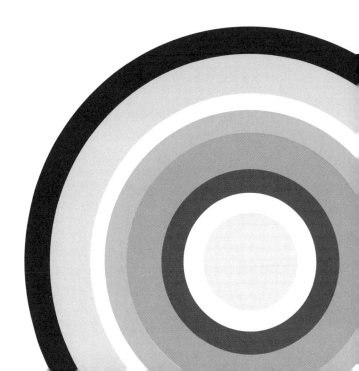

Nature has provided us with a powerhouse of energy-giving foods, so when you're dashing round the supermarket or snatching a quick lunch break, do yourself a favour – avoid those high-fat, high-sugar fast foods and swap them for my top twelve energy superfoods.

energy superfood 1

baked potatoes

Rich in fibre, vitamins B and C, potassium and with no fat. Don't add mayonnaise, butter or cream cheese but serve with spicy tomato sauce and green salad.

energy superfood 2

bananas

Nature's miracle fast food. They're not fattening and are full of essential nutrients like potassium, zinc, iron, vitamin B6 and folic acid. They will also give you instant energy. Bananas are easily digested and their high potassium content helps prevent cramp.

beans

energy superfood 3

Good old baked beans, like all their bean and pulse relatives, provide slow-release energy and are rich in protein, carbohydrates and soluble fibre. Tinned beans are fine, but rinse well to remove the salt. Use in salads, soups and casseroles for a real vitality boost.

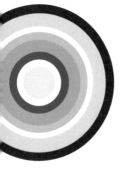
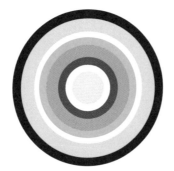
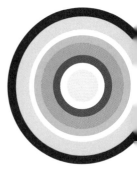

vegetable, bean and barley soup

An amazing combination of instant and slow-release energy, this typical peasant dish is cheap, filling and nourishing.

45g pot barley
4 carrots, finely sliced
1 turnip, chopped
2 leeks, sliced
2 stalks celery, sliced
1 onion, chopped
1 tbsp tomato purée
1 litre water
1 x 400g can kidney beans, drained and rinsed

Bring the first 7 ingredients to the boil in the water. Simmer for 45 minutes until tender. Add the kidney beans and cook for a further 5 minutes. Ladle into soup bowls and serve immediately.

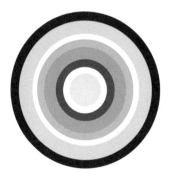

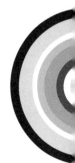

energy superfood 4

pasta

For instant energy that will also keep you going for three or four hours. Add tuna, tomato sauce, stir-fried vegetables or, as millions of Italians do every day, a drizzle of olive oil and some finely chopped garlic. Go easy on the Parmesan.

green pasta with tuna fish

450g spinach tagliatelle
2 tbsp extra-virgin
  olive oil
4 large spring onions,
  chopped (including
  the green parts)
1 x 400g can tuna
4 large tomatoes,
  roughly chopped

Cook the pasta in a large saucepan of boiling water according to the packet instructions. Meanwhile, heat the oil in a saucepan and sauté the spring onions gently until soft. Add the tuna and warm through gently. Drain the pasta and return to the pan. Mix the fish and onion mixture, with the tomatoes, into the pasta and serve.

energy superfood 5

rice

Very low in fat, with protein, B vitamins and, especially if it's brown, masses of slow-release energy. Brown rice takes a little longer to cook than white but provides more of all the nutrients. Eat it hot for your evening meal and take the leftovers to work in a rice salad.

brown rice risotto with sun-dried tomatoes

Strictly speaking, you cook risotto by stirring the stock in gradually over about 30 minutes. But this dish is more boiled rice with vegetables than risotto, which makes it easier. It's also extremely high in energy and delicious hot or cold.

3 tbsp rapeseed oil
1 onion, finely chopped
2 garlic cloves, finely chopped
225g brown rice
200g sun-dried tomatoes
4 tomatoes, roughly chopped
800ml vegetable stock
3 tbsp Cheddar cheese, grated
10 leaves basil, roughly torn

Heat the oil in a large non-stick frying pan and sauté the onion and garlic gently until just turning golden. Add the rice, sun-dried tomatoes snipped to the size of a raisin, fresh tomatoes and stock. Simmer for 40 minutes, adding extra stock or water, if necessary. Stir in the cheese, sprinkle on the basil and serve.

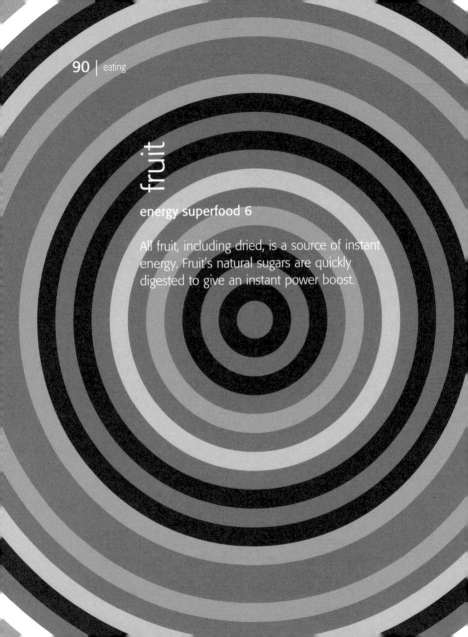

fruit

energy superfood 6

All fruit, including dried, is a source of instant energy. Fruit's natural sugars are quickly digested to give an instant power boost.

fresh fruit kebabs

Simple, impressive and wonderfully healthy as part of your detox regime.

4 wooden skewers
1 small pineapple, peeled and cubed
about 100g large seedless black grapes
1 apple, cored and cubed
2 pears, cored and cubed
4 tbsp runny honey
4 pinches ground cloves

Soak the skewers in water for 30 minutes before using to prevent burning. Preheat the grill to high and line a grill pan with foil. Make sure the pieces of fruit are roughly the same size and thread them on to the skewers. Put the kebabs on the foil-lined grill pan, drizzle with the honey and sprinkle with the ground cloves. Cook under a very hot grill for 2 minutes, then serve.

sweetcorn

energy superfood 7

Seldom on the list of healthy foods, but one of my favourites and a great energy booster. Add to salads and soups, or eat with a modest amount of butter and lots of black pepper.

oats

energy superfood 8

The cheapest and best breakfast of all, offering B vitamins for your nervous system, vitamin E for your heart and skin, and slow-release energy, which will keep you going till lunchtime without giving you the mid-morning munchies. Always start the day with porridge or muesli.

lentils

energy superfood 9

Very high in protein and containing lots of iron
to prevent anaemia and stop you feeling tired.
Lentils also contain B vitamins for memory and
mental faculties and are a great source of fat-free,
energy-giving calories. Delicious in traditional
Indian dhal or on their own with meat dishes or
in salads.

lentil and barley pilaff

125g pot barley
600ml vegetable stock
225g brown lentils
4 tbsp olive oil
1 carrot, finely chopped
1 stick celery, finely
  chopped
2 onions, sliced
1 tbsp freshly chopped
  parsley leaves
175g live natural
  yoghurt

Wash the barley, soak in cold water to cover for 1 hour and drain. Put the stock into a large saucepan, add the barley and simmer, covered, for 45 minutes or until tender. Meanwhile, cook the lentils according to the packet instructions (this normally takes 30–40 minutes). Heat 1 tbsp of the oil in a frying pan and gently sauté the carrot, celery and half the onions for 4 minutes. Mix with the barley and lentils and keep warm in a 180°C/350°F/Gas 4 oven. Heat the rest of the oil in a frying pan and fry the remaining onion. Serve the pilaff garnished with the onion rings and parsley and with the yoghurt on the side.

energy superfood 10

nuts and seeds

Not chocolate-covered, not salted, just natural. Delicious and rich in protein and minerals, particularly zinc and selenium, they offer a gentle, continual energy release, which makes them perfect to carry around and nibble on at any time of the day.

buckwheat

energy superfood 11

You may never have heard of it and you probably haven't knowingly tasted it, but buckwheat is used to make those wonderful French, Dutch and Belgian pancakes as well as the ones served with Chinese duck. It's not a cereal, but a relative of rhubarb, and as well as providing loads of energy, it's great for the circulation and helps reduce high blood pressure.

bread

energy superfood 12

The staff of life, but because people think it's fattening, we don't eat nearly enough of it. Aim for at least four or five slices a day. Wholemeal is of course best, but there are now so many wonderful breads available that you can mix and match. Bread contains masses of energy, virtually no fat – unless you smother it with butter – lots of B vitamins and everything you need to keep you on the go. Never eat slimming bread, low-calorie bread, or the cheap sliced white bread that's like cotton wool.

my easy bread

Most commercial bread contains added chemicals as well as far too much salt, both of which are highly undesirable. The answer is to make your own.

700g stoneground organic wholemeal bread flour

1 x 7g sachet easy-blend dried yeast

2 tsp extra-virgin olive oil, plus extra for oiling

1 tsp dark molasses, muscovado sugar or honey

$1/2$ tsp salt

600ml warm water

2 tbsp sunflower seeds (optional)

Mix the flour and yeast in a large bowl. Dissolve the oil, molasses and salt in the water. Make a well in the flour and add the molasses mixture and sunflower seeds, if using. Mix with a wooden spoon, then knead until the dough forms a ball. Place in a warmed, lightly oiled 1kg tin, cover with a damp tea towel and leave in a warm place for 40 minutes or until the dough has risen almost to the top. Meanwhile, heat the oven to 200°C/400°F/Gas 6. Bake for 40 minutes, until the loaf sounds hollow when you tap the bottom. Transfer to a wire rack to cool completely.

my top five energy superherbs

When you're eating my top twelve energy superfoods, don't forget that natural herbs can help your energy levels too. Add these five to your cooking for a double dose of energy. You can never have too much.

rosemary

energy superherb 1

This versatile herb is a rich source of volatile essential oils and flavonoids, which are extremely energising as well as mood-enhancing. It also boosts your brain power and memory. It's perfect in soups, salads and pasta dishes and is ideal for flavouring oils, vinegars and marinades.

grilled lamb cutlets with rosemary

4 lamb cutlets
6 tbsp extra-virgin
  olive oil
2 cloves garlic, finely
  chopped
4 tbsp fresh rosemary,
  very finely chopped
  leaves

Trim any excess fat off the cutlets. Mix the oil, garlic and rosemary together in a large shallow dish. Add the cutlets and turn to coat in the marinade. Cover and leave to marinate in the fridge for 2 hours, turning occasionally. Preheat the grill to high. Remove the cutlets from the marinade, leaving some of the liquid still clinging, and cook under the preheated grill for 2–3 minutes on each side. Serve immediately.

energy superherb 2

sage

This gives a real power boost to your energy levels, but only if you use the right variety. The most important constituent for energy is the natural substance thujone, but there's virtually none of that in the commonly sold Spanish sage. For the richest source and most potent energy booster, use purple sage, which is particularly good for women as it helps even out those hormone imbalances that are the cause of low energy levels. Add sage to almost any savoury dish you like or use it to make a tea.

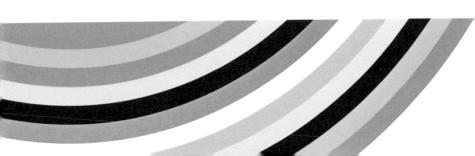

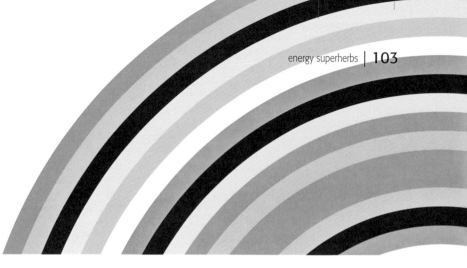

energy superherb 3

marjoram

This is the ideal energizing herb to accompany oily fish, casseroles or meat dishes. It contains anti-viral and anti-bacterial eugenol and energy-boosting estragole. Often called sweet marjoram, it's the most potent of this family of plants and is closely related to oregano, hence its botanical name, *Oreganum majorana*.

lavender

energy superherb 4

Everyone knows that lavender oil is good for headaches, but few people make use of this wonderful herb in cooking. It contains more than 40 plant chemicals, with masses of energy-boosting volatile oils, protective coumarins and flavonoids. Use the flowers to make a delicious and refreshing tea, add them to biscuits, cakes or ice creams or, surprisingly, use them together with the finely chopped leaves in rich meat-based soups, casseroles and stews.

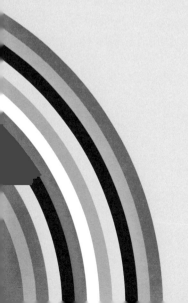

energy superherb 5

bay

This is a rather abused herb which is often overlooked for its valuable medicinal properties. A rich source of energising laurenolide, bay is also good for chest infections and depression as well as for bringing on delayed periods. In addition to the traditional use in savoury dishes, try it in all milk-based puddings as it enhances their flavours in a surprising way. It really is worth growing your own bay as the fresh leaves have a much more subtle and delicate taste than the dried.

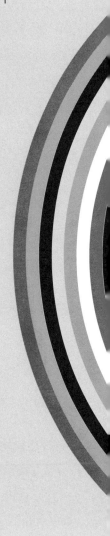

parsley

super skin special

You'll find that parsley is wonderful for the skin. It's a gentle diuretic, which helps the body get rid of fluid, and it's also rich in vitamins A and C as well as being a reasonable source of iron. Make it into parsley tea (see page 17) and drink a glass every day.

ten-minute mussels

50g unsalted butter
4 shallots, very finely
chopped
2 cloves garlic, peeled
and very finely
chopped
1 red chilli, deseeded
and finely chopped
5 tbsp parsley leaves,
freshly chopped
$\frac{1}{2}$ bottle dry white
wine
2kg mussels, washed,
beards removed and
any open shells
discarded

Melt the butter in a pan
large enough to hold all
the mussels and sauté the
shallots, garlic and chilli
gently. Add the chopped
parsley, pour in the wine
and bring to the boil. Add
the mussels. Cover the pan
and cook over a medium
heat for 5 minutes until the
shells open. Discard any
that don't open. Using a
slotted spoon, put the
mussels into serving bowls.
Bring the rest of the liquid
to a very fast boil for 3
minutes. Pour over the
mussels and serve.

cloves

super skin special

Cloves are a great aid to digestion and also help in the treatment of irritable bowel syndrome – and anything that improves your digestive output will mean better skin and clearer eyes. Use it when cooking fruits as well as in stews and casseroles made from lamb, game or venison.

spiced baked apples

The simple addition of ground almonds and raisins adds valuable energy-giving calories and a host of other essential nutrients to this simple dessert.

2 tbsp ground almonds
1 tbsp raisins
1 tbsp orange juice
4 cooking apples, washed, cored and with the bottom 1cm of the core replaced
4 cloves
50g unsalted butter
1 tbsp brown sugar
4 pinches freshly ground nutmeg

Preheat the oven to 190°C/375°F/Gas 5. Mix together the almonds, raisins and orange juice. Spoon into the cored cavities of the apples. Top each one with a clove. Use half the butter to grease a large ovenproof dish and the other half to smear over the apple skins. Place the apples in the dish, sprinkle over the sugar and nutmeg and bake in the preheated oven for 25 minutes.

basil

super skin special

This is a superb remedy for tension and anxiety headaches – a common cause of frowning and wrinkles – but as well as that, it also has a gentle calming and soothing action which will help you relax and unwind. It's also useful for improving irregular periods.

one-pot pasta with vegetables and pesto

Another quick, easy and inexpensive meal that takes minimum effort and gives maximum benefit. As well as the skin-friendly nutrients in the vegetables and the pesto, there's added value from the mood-enhancing essential oils in the basil, which is what pesto is usually made from.

400g spaghetti
75g french beans, finely chopped
2 courgettes, finely diced
3 new potatoes, very finely diced
4 tbsp pesto sauce
3 tbsp Parmesan cheese, freshly grated

Bring a large saucepan of water to the boil and add the spaghetti and vegetables. They will all be just tender at the same time, about 6 minutes. Drain, reserving 2 tsp of the water and mix this in a bowl with the pesto. Mix the pesto with the drained pasta and vegetables. Add the Parmesan and serve immediately.

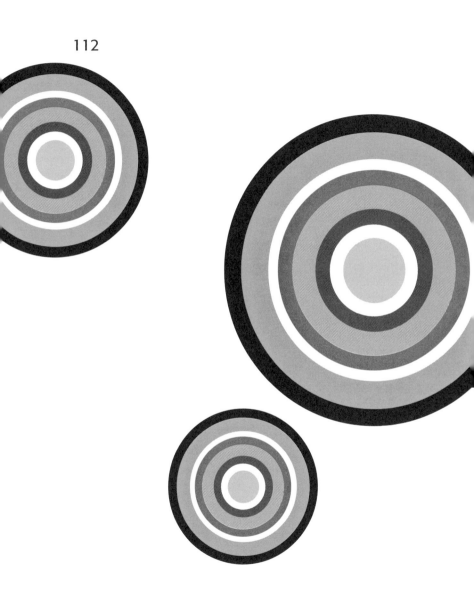

arthritis tip

Stave off arthritis by eating oily fish three times a week.

menopause years

Drink at least 250ml soya milk, or eat a portion of tofu or soya beans each day. These contain plant hormones that counteract the problems of the menopause and protect against osteoporosis.

natural plant hormones

The natural plant hormones that can be extracted from soya beans, red clover and other plant material can be of major benefit. They are particularly important in the treatment of acne, skin problems relate to irregular periods, hormone imbalance, polycystic ovarian syndrome, adult acne, and at all stages of women's menopausal years – pre-, during and post-menopause.

tofu, vegetable and cashew nut stir-fry

Tofu is also known as soya-bean curd. This recipe will provide you with natural plant hormones from the tofu, antibacterial sulphur from the cabbage, masses of vitamin A from the carrots and more than your day's requirement of vitamin C.

3 tbsp olive oil
250g tofu, drained and
  cubed
1 onion, finely chopped
1 green pepper,
  deseeded and cubed
1cm fresh root ginger,
  grated
1 stalk celery, finely
  sliced
2 medium carrots,
  finely sliced
1/2 shredded cabbage
100g mushrooms,
  wiped and sliced
125g cashew nuts
200ml vegetable stock
1 tsp soy sauce

Heat the oil in a preheated wok, add the tofu and fry gently until golden brown. Remove from the wok with a slotted spoon and reserve. Add the onion, green pepper, ginger and celery and sauté gently until soft. Add the carrots and cabbage and sauté for 4 minutes longer. Add the mushrooms and cashew nuts and cook for a further 1 minute. Pour in the stock and cover and simmer until the vegetables are soft. Just before serving, add the fried tofu and the soy sauce.

the wonder of fish oils

The essential fatty acids (EFAs) in fish oils are vital for the growth and development of the brain and nervous system, but many of us do not eat as much fish as our parents or grandparents did.

help! I'm vegetarian

If you're a vegetarian or vegan or are allergic to fish, then you should use flaxseeds or flaxseed oil instead of fish oils, though they aren't as beneficial. If you're vegetarian or vegan and are planning a pregnancy or are pregnant or breastfeeding, I really do urge you to take a fish-oil supplement, if not for your own sake, then for that of your baby.

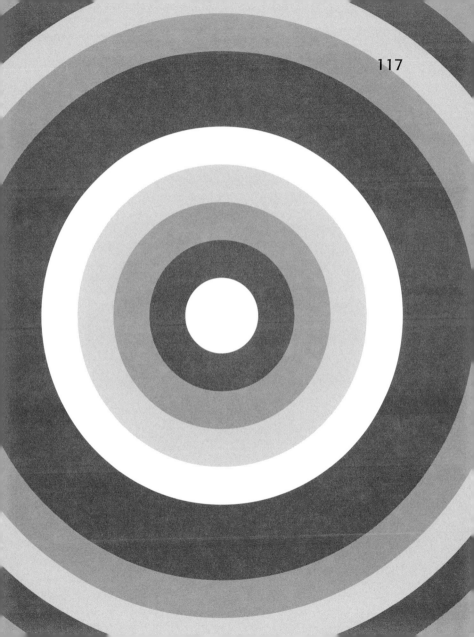

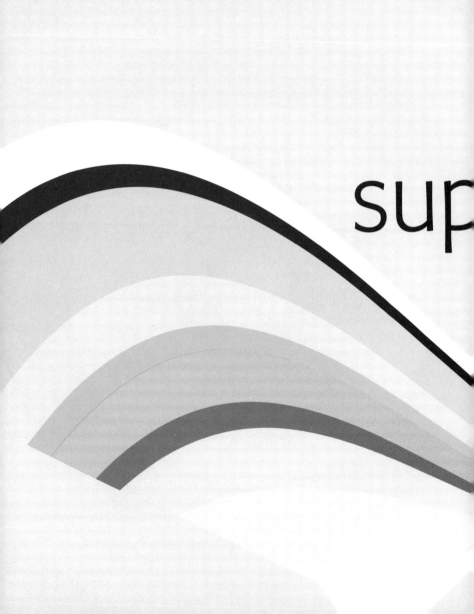

sup

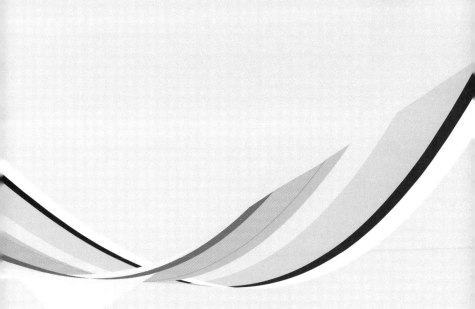
olementing

six natural supplements for permanent health protection

For permanent health protection against all the things our bodies have to contend with – toxic residues in food, environmental pollutants at home, stress, even the air we breathe – these six natural supplements are the added extras you need.

1 saw palmetto

The North American Indians were the first to discover the benefits of this small palm tree. Chewing its berries not only gave their men Gladiator-style muscles, it also did wonders for their love lives. Now, a thousand years on, it's the most effective natural remedy for reducing an enlarged prostate.

2 green tea

Three to five cups of Japanese or Chinese green tea a day could protect you from many forms of cancer, particularly cancer of the throat. Scientists first noticed the benefits in Japan, where they drink loads of the stuff. Now, America's leading cancer organisation has provided evidence that chemicals called catechins in the tea prevent the growth of tumours.

hypericum 3

Feeling down in the dumps isn't a twenty-first century phenomenon. Hypericum, also known as St John's wort, is a pretty garden plant. It has been called 'the sunshine herb' and has been used to treat psychological problems since the Middle Ages. The most recent research shows that it can treat mild to moderate depression in 70 per cent of sufferers without any side effects or risk of addiction. I've seen patients improve dramatically in two to four weeks.

Despite its unlikely nickname – its real name is the more wordy *Harpagophytum procumbens* – this African desert plant brings enormous relief to people suffering from arthritis and rheumatism. It's known as Devil's Claw because of the vicious hooks on its fruits, which stick to the feet of animals or humans. I know because I trod on a few when I was out digging for it with the bushmen in the Namibian desert. They've been using it as an anti-inflammatory medicine for centuries.

4
devil's claw

5 selenium

+ vitamins a, c and e

This is a vital combination of powerful antioxidants and should always be taken during periods of increased stress, before and after surgery, after any major trauma or serious illness, and before and during prolonged periods of physical exertion. The combination provides permanent protection against damage to individual body cells and can specifically help to prevent heart disease as well as breast and prostate cancers.

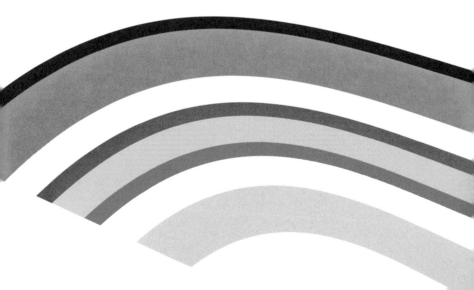

6 glucosamine sulphate

Used to help relieve joint pain and to repair
cartilage, glucosamine first came to my attention
when Olympic swimmer David Wilkie told me
about it. He'd been given it in America. When
we're young we naturally produce enough
glucosamine to repair cartilage damage. The
trouble starts when, as in David's case, we put
extra strain on our joints, or when we get older.

vitamin a

This is necessary for building new skin tissue and healing skin damage. Fortunately, your body is clever enough to manufacture vitamin A from betacarotene, so make sure you eat an average portion from this list every single day – liver (not if you're pregnant), carrots, spinach, broccoli, sweet potatoes, cantaloupe melon, nectarines and apricots.

apricot and almond crumble

Don't feel guilty about enjoying this delicious pudding. After all, feeling good is a major factor in looking good, and enjoyment of any sort helps you feel good. On top of that, apricots are a major source of vitamin A, almonds provide vitamin E and essential minerals, and oats are rich in the B vitamins. So this is a really sweet treat.

50g unsalted butter, cut
   into small cubes
50g apricots, stoned
   and halved
2 tbsp demerara sugar
175g porridge oats
50g ground almonds
1 tbsp runny honey
75g flaked almonds

Preheat the oven to 200°C/400°F/Gas 6. Use about half the butter to grease a pie dish. Add the apricots, sugar and 2 tbsp of water. Mix the oats and ground almonds together in a bowl and sprinkle over the top. Drizzle with the honey. Scatter over the flaked almonds and dot with the rest of the butter. Bake in the preheated oven for 20 minutes.

This is the nutrient that's so very important for the health of the skin and as a protective antioxidant. Get your daily requirements by eating avocados, asparagus, extra-virgin olive oil, cod-liver oil, wheatgerm oil, almonds and all seeds, for example sunflower seeds and sesame seeds.

vitamin **e**

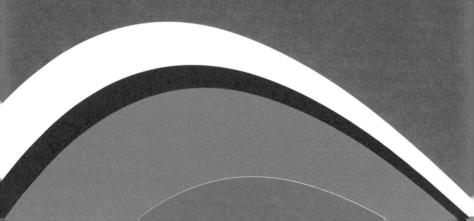

baked cod with sesame seeds

It's the sesame seeds that make this simple dish different. Like all seeds, sesame seeds are rich in vitamin E. They'll also give you a massive energy boost.

4 cod steaks
2 eggs, beaten
110g sesame seeds

Preheat the oven to 160°C/325°F/Gas 3. Dip the fish into the eggs, then into the sesame seeds. Put on a large baking sheet and cook in the preheated oven for 20 minutes.

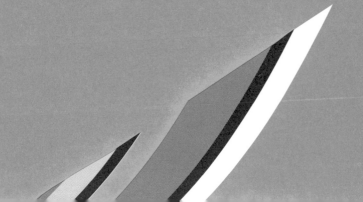

b vitamins

These are essential, especially for the nervous system, while vitamin B12 also prevents pernicious anaemia. The B vitamins are found in yeast, wholegrain cereals, chickpeas, liver and all meat. Vitamin B12 is also in eggs, cheese, yoghurt, yeast extracts and beer. Two teaspoons of liver contain more than a day's B vitamins requirement.

quick chickpea casserole

Cheap, filling, easy to use but much ignored, chickpeas are an excellent food. Apart from their cleansing fibre and B vitamins, they also contain minerals essential for maintaining the structure and elasticity of the skin.

4 tbsp olive oil
1 onion, finely chopped
3 cloves garlic, finely
   chopped
1 x 400g can tomatoes
1 x 400g can chickpeas
450g frozen mixed
   vegetables
1 sachet bouquet garni
900ml stock
2 tbsp parsley, freshly
   chopped leaves

Heat the olive oil in a large saucepan and sauté the onion and garlic gently until just soft. Pour in the tomatoes with their juice and bring to a simmer. Meanwhile, drain and rinse the chickpeas. Add the chickpeas, mixed vegetables, bouquet garni sachet and stock to the onion and garlic mixture and simmer for 15 minutes. Sprinkle with the chopped parsley and serve.

folic acid

This is a vital B vitamin that prevents birth defects and heart disease. It's in vegetables and cereals. Meet your daily needs with 100g of spinach or 170g of either potatoes, Brussels sprouts, chickpeas, broccoli, kale or asparagus.

This is needed by every cell but isn't stored by the body. Ensure you get enough by making soups or gravies with the water you've cooked your vegetables in. A large baked potato, a portion of vegetable curry, a dozen dried apricots, a herring or a mackerel, a couple of bananas, a watercress salad or a handful of raisins, will make up for any deficiencies.

potassium

This vitamin is essential for bone strength. Oily fish, margarine and eggs are the most important sources – 40g of herring or kipper, 60g of mackerel, 85g of tinned salmon or 140g of tinned sardines will each provide your daily requirement.

vitamin **d**

pan-fried liver

Liver is the organ that stores agricultural chemicals, so buy organic whenever you can. It's the richest source of vitamin A, contains the most easily absorbed iron and supplies lots of vitamins B12 and D. This is a quick, easy and healthy recipe – but not if you're pregnant as the huge amount of vitamin A could damage your baby.

4 tbsp rapeseed oil
50g unsalted butter
1 large onion, finely chopped
4 thin rashers unsmoked back bacon, cut in two lengthways
700g calves' liver, thinly sliced
5 tbsp sherry
4 tbsp parsley, finely chopped leaves

Heat the oil and butter in a saucepan and sauté the onion and bacon until just turning gold. Remove with a slotted spoon and reserve. Add the liver to the pan and cook until just turning brown, about 1 minute on each side. Return the onion and bacon to the pan, pour in the sherry and heat until bubbling. Stir in the parsley and serve immediately.

This is essential for bones. Find virtually all you need in 10g of whitebait, 10g of cheese, 10g of tinned sardines, half a litre of milk (skimmed, semi-skimmed or whole), or 40g of tofu.

calcium

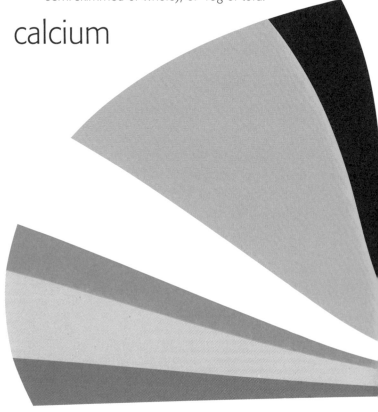

posh cauliflower cheese with pasta

The pasta, oil and cheese in this different type of traditional cauliflower cheese give you masses of energy. And as a bonus, there's the calcium in the cheese and plenty of cancer-protective nutrients in the cauliflower.

275g sun-dried tomato spaghetti
1 cauliflower, cut into small florets
4 tbsp extra-virgin olive oil
1 large onion, finely chopped
75ml dry white wine
2 eggs, beaten
3 tbsp Parmesan cheese, freshly grated
4 tbsp fresh basil, roughly torn leaves

Cook the pasta according to the instructions on the packet. Meanwhile, blanch the cauliflower in boiling water for 2 minutes, then drain. Heat the olive oil in a large saucepan and sauté the onion gently. Add the cauliflower and wine and simmer gently. Mix together the eggs, cheese and half the basil. Drain the cooked pasta and add to the cauliflower. Pour over the egg mixture, stirring continuously over a gentle heat until the egg scrambles. Sprinkle over the extra basil leaves and serve.

magnesium

This is essential for every cell and is important to the way calcium and potassium are utilised by your body. You'll find magnesium in cereals, nuts, green vegetables, beans, peas, millet and in wholemeal bread.

iron

This is vital for the blood, and the best sources are meat and offal, though whitebait, mussels, cockles and winkles also contain large amounts. Vegetable sources are not so easily absorbed. Get more than your recommended daily dose from eating 60g of cockles, 140g of liver or 170g of mussels. You can also get valuable amounts of iron from a portion of dahl, a portion of vegetable curry, a portion of beans or a portion of dark-green vegetables.

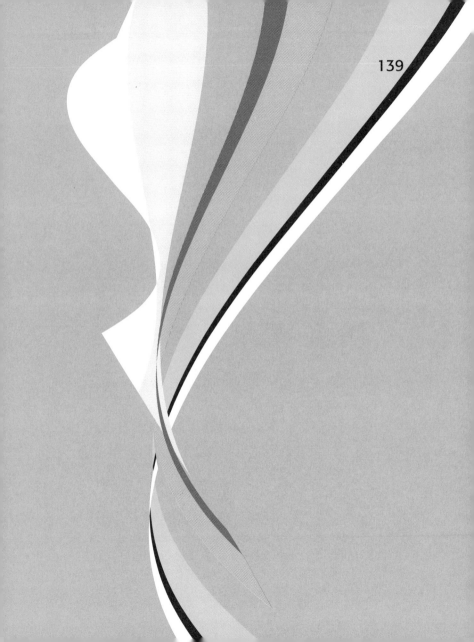

zinc

Make sure that your complement of zinc is up to the mark by adding red meat, shellfish, sardines, poultry, kidney beans, yeast, nuts and pumpkin seeds to your shopping list. By the way, zinc is also vital for the manufacture of sperm. The richest source of all is the oyster – Casanova was reputed to eat seventy oysters a day!

sage burgers

These are a highly nutritious alternative to meat-based burgers, and with the bonus that they contain no saturated fat. Added to that, they are rich in skin-friendly minerals, especially zinc and selenium, and have lots of fibre, which encourages good digestion. The nuts also provide radiance-enhancing vitamin E.

225g mixed nuts
110g wholemeal breadcrumbs
about 125ml sunflower oil
1 medium onion, very finely chopped
300ml vegetable stock
2 tsp yeast extract
6 sage leaves, finely chopped
4 tbsp wholemeal flour, for dusting

Grind the nuts and breadcrumbs together. Heat 2 tbsp of the oil in a saucepan and sauté the onion gently until soft. Heat the stock and yeast extract together in a saucepan until blended. Mix the ground nuts, breadcrumbs and onion together, adding enough stock and yeast extract mixture to make a good consistency. Shape into 4 burgers and dust with the flour. Heat the rest of the oil in a large pan and shallow-fry the burgers for 4 minutes on each side.

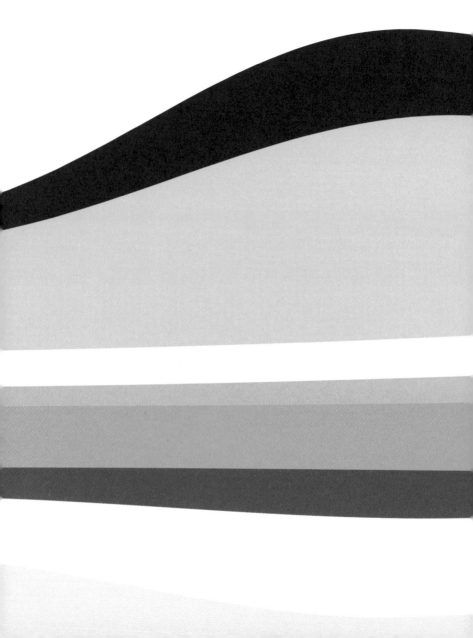

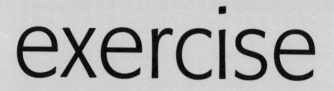

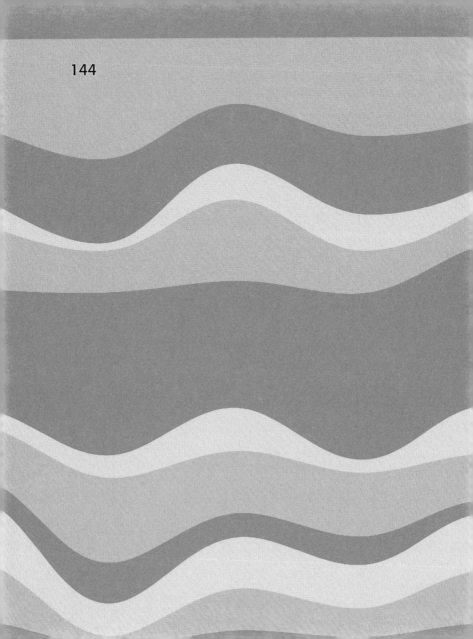

144

four reasons to exercise

1 Exercise builds muscle strength, which improves posture, prevents backache and reduces the pain of arthritis.

2 Exercise improves the health and efficiency of lungs, circulation and the heart. And as your heart grows stronger, it's able to pump more blood with fewer beats and less effort, which reduces the strain on the heart itself and prolongs its healthy active life.

3 Exercise boosts your natural immunity and increases the body's resistance to disease and infection.

4 Exercise makes you feel good emotionally as physical activity releases mood-boosting hormones in the brain.

fit to exercise?

Before starting any exercise programme you must assess your own fitness. If you are overweight and over 40 and you've hardly moved a muscle since you left school, seek professional advice before you start. And the same is true if you've ever been told that you have high blood pressure or heart disease. To help you decide how you stand, answer the following questions truthfully, then add up the number of yeses.

1 Are you over 40?

2 Is it more than 5 years since you took regular exercise?

3 Do you regularly get home and fall asleep in front of the TV?

4 Do you have any joint disease or deformity?

5 Are you more than 7 kilos overweight?

6 Do you ever get dizzy or faint?

7 Do you smoke?

8 Do you feel ill if you have had to run for the train?

9 Do you get out of breath easily?

10 Do you have a problem sleeping?

11 Have you ever had a serious back problem?

12 Do you drink more than 1.5 litres of beer, 3 glasses of wine or 3 spirits daily?

0–3 yeses
Good, but start exercising today.

3–6 yeses
Just in time; start gently and persevere.

6–12 yeses
You may not make it to the gym! Get some advice before you start.

question how do I make exercise part
of my life?

answer The most important thing is to choose an activity
you enjoy and one that's appropriate to your age,
ability and general health. It doesn't matter if it's
walking the dog, playing bowls, windsurfing or
riding a bike – half an hour, three times a week
will improve your health permanently.

did you know that….?

….fitness is a combination of strength, mobility and stamina and ideally you need all three. There's no point being strong if you can't bend down to tie your shoelace or extremely mobile if you can't keep up with your children on a five-kilometre walk.

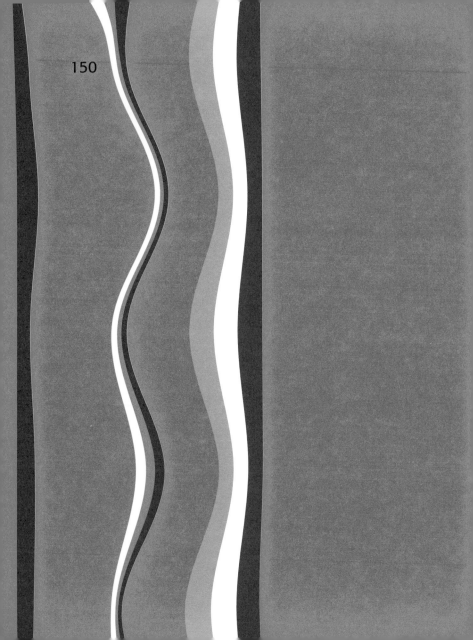

150

be a water baby

Swimming is excellent for getting mobile, especially if you spend most of your working life at a desk or in front of a computer, where poor posture results in a shortening of muscles, tendons and ligaments and a gradual loss of joint mobility. When you're swimming, 70 per cent of your body weight is supported by the water so you'll find that stiff hips and knees, rigid backs and immobile neck and shoulder joints all move far more easily. And an added bonus is that swimming can substantially improve your breathing, so it's a particularly valuable form of exercise for asthmatics.

You can combine straightforward swimming with aquarobics – specially designed exercises to do in the pool. Initially it's best to learn these in a class. Once you've mastered them, you can combine them with your regular swimming sessions.

the three stages of exercise

1 Warm-ups will gently stretch the muscles, speed up the circulation and increase your pulse rate. They also start the release of the body's feel-good hormones that put you in the right frame of mind for exercise. Your warm-up has got to last a minimum of five minutes and it's just as important if you're a regular athlete as it is if you're starting from scratch.

2 The endurance stage of your programme should last for 20–30 minutes, during which you push your heart rate up and keep it there. You shouldn't end up gasping for breath but as your stamina increases, you'll need to increase the length of exercise or its intensity. In the early stages, it's better to exercise less vigorously but for slightly longer periods.

3 The cooling-down phase is vital as it allows your heart rate and breathing to return to normal gradually, while the combination of stretching and alternate walking and jogging lets your muscles cool down slowly. You need at least six minutes in this phase.

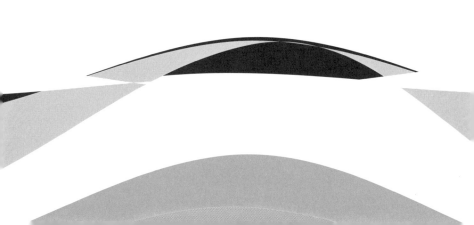

don't obsess

Whatever you do, remember that your exercise regime should be fun and you mustn't allow it to become an obsession.

mix and match

You may find you prefer to stick to one activity, like tennis, though you'll get a better balance of strength and mobility if you do a range of different sports. A session in the gym, a session of your favourite sport and a swim is a great weekly combination. With a bit of experimentation you'll soon find what fits best with your personal preferences, work and lifestyle.

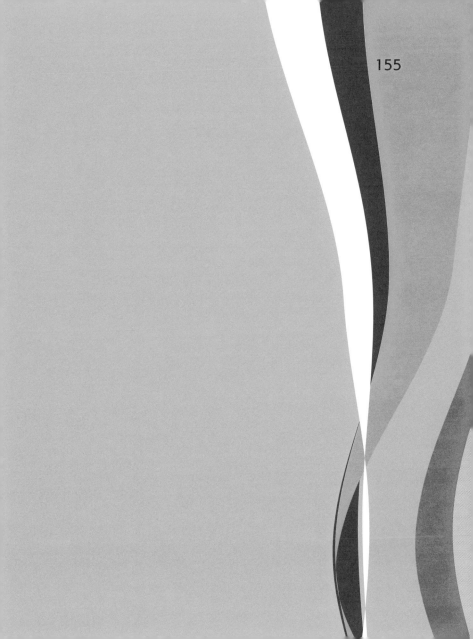

when not to exercise

- If you have a heavy cold or a raised temperature.

- If you have or develop pain in the chest.

- If you have persistent joint or muscle pains for which you haven't had professional advice.

- If the weather is either extremely hot or extremely cold.

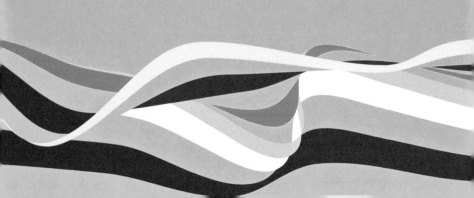

check your heart rate

Most adult men and women have a resting heart rate of 60–80 beats per minute. Find yours by pressing your wrist on the thumb side, counting the beats for 15 seconds, then multiplying by four to find the rate per minute. When you exercise, you should aim to push your heart rate up to the level recommended in the table below.

age	beats per min
20	138 – 158
25	137 – 156
30	135 – 154
35	134 – 153
40	132 – 151
45	131 – 150
50	129 – 147
55	127 – 146
60	126 – 144
65	125 – 142
70	123 – 141
75	122 – 139
80	120 – 138
85	119 – 136

time for a reward

Take a shower or bath to cool down and relax your tired muscles after exercise. Take your time, don't rush – and enjoy it. This is a reward for you and your muscles.

don't stretch to breaking point

When warming up and cooling down, make sure you do the stretching exercises slowly and gradually. Any short jerky movements will make your muscles contract and be more liable to damage.

new to exercise and feeling stiff?

Don't worry if you feel a bit stiff to begin with. Your body simply isn't accustomed to exercise. These aches and pains will stop as you gradually get fitter.

question do I need sports drinks and
energy boosters when I exercise?

answer Keeping well hydrated is extremely important, but
stick to plain water and avoid fizzy drinks as these
can make you bloated and uncomfortable. Unless
you're working extremely hard, you have no need
whatsoever of sports drinks or energy boosters.
A banana or some dried fruits an hour before you
exercise, plenty of water during your activity and
more water or diluted orange juice afterwards are
quite adequate.

two exercise no-nos

1 Train not strain, so build up your exercise gradually.

2 Don't be competitive. This is not the time to try to keep up with a friend who's been doing aerobics classes for years, or to challenge the new office junior to a game of squash when you haven't played since you were 20.

take your partners

I've learned from experience with my patients that it's far more effective to do your fitness routine with a partner. It's a lot more fun and if you know someone is waiting for you at the gym, the park or the swimming pool, you're more likely to keep going.

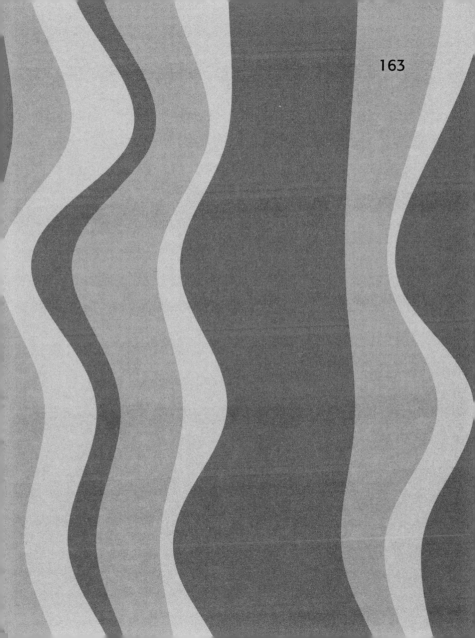

163

did you know that....?

....the old adage 'use it or lose it' is just as applicable to mental processes as it is to your back, leg or any other muscles. To really generate revitalising mental energy you have to make your brain cells work, and work hard at that. You'll only achieve this by constantly challenging your mental abilities and always seeking to push a little beyond what you think you can achieve.

two tips for improving short-term memory

1 Play Kim's Game – an old stand-by of the worldwide Boy Scout movement – this is one of the great memory improvers. Have someone place 20 different objects on a tray, cover them with a cloth and then allow you to look at the objects for just 60 seconds. Replace the cloth, then try to write down as many objects as you can remember. Initially you may struggle to remember more than a handful, but with regular practice you'll be amazed at how quickly you'll be able to recall almost all of them.

2 Learning by heart – you can improve both short- and long-term memory by learning poetry, speeches from plays, or quotations from well-known books. To make this work, you have to do it on a regular basis, so every night before you go to bed, commit a few lines to memory and make sure you can repeat them the next morning, and the morning after that, and a month after that. You may not have tried to memorise a poem since your schooldays, but the mental energy it generates will mean a permanent improvement. You may find you can't manage more than five or six lines to begin with but, before you know it, your party piece will be the opening prologue from Shakespeare's *Henry V*.

that's mental

Practise mental arithmetic for a few minutes every single day to prevent a decline in your short-term memory function. Try these mental maths exercises. The answers are on page 304.

1   10 x 10 + 12

2 $\dfrac{7 \times 8 \times 2 - 2}{10}$

3 $\dfrac{13 + 7}{5 \times 12}$

4 $\dfrac{23 \times 4 - 50}{7}$

5   17 + 14 + 106 + 33 − 27

6   109 + 72 + 226 + 593

7   10,425 + 8,659 + 28,694 x 100

seven things you may not know about yoga

1 Yoga has existed in India for thousands of years.

2 It is ideal for people of any age.

3 In the West, it is mostly associated with certain postures that promote mobility and flexibility and that also have therapeutic benefits.

4 The concentration required helps eliminate stress and anxiety, so reducing the levels of adrenaline circulating in the bloodstream. This helps to lower blood pressure and reduce the strain on the heart and blood vessels.

5 Combining the postures with traditional yoga breathing helps establish patterns of profound relaxation and inner peace which can combat the lunatic pace of life that most of us live at in the twenty-first century.

6 If you haven't exercised for a while, yoga's a safe way to start gently stretching and mobilising your joints, muscles and ligaments without the risk of injury.

7 You can learn the simple poses from books and videos but it's always best to learn from an experienced teacher who will ensure that you achieve the positions with the minimum effort and without risk of injury. For maximum benefit, once you're familiar with the postures, you need to practise on a daily basis.

three things you may not know about weight-bearing exercise

1 The most important thing you can do to combat osteoporosis is weight-bearing exercise.

2 Although most bone building goes on during the late teens, it's never too late to encourage your bones to strengthen themselves.

3 You can get your exercise in any way that you enjoy, but you have to have your weight on your feet, so swimming and cycling don't count. A brisk 20-minute walk four times a week is all you need.

seven things you may not know about alexander technique

1 Alexander was a struggling actor who discovered that his voice problems were caused by tension and bad posture. He developed his system to deal with these and over the years Alexander technique has become hugely popular with dancers, musicians and performers of all kinds.

2 It offers a process of physical re-education that corrects the postural bad habits you've developed during your life. You will gradually come to feel uncomfortable with your bad old postural habits and will recognise what feels good and healthy.

3 It can help with many conditions such as asthma, migraine, high blood pressure, backache and bowel problems.

4 It also has a positive effect on your circulation and breathing. This will improve the oxygen-carrying ability of your blood.

5 Alexander is one technique that you cannot learn from books, videos or from the internet.

6 An Alexander teacher will gently realign your body to re-establish the perfect relationship between your head, neck and trunk.

7 The technique also focuses on discovering how to use the minimum muscular effort required to achieve any single task.

wellbeing

stay positive

People who see their glass as half empty are often those who find it impossible to take responsibility for their own actions. They believe the grass is always greener on the other side of the fence and think it's always someone else's fault they didn't get that promotion. They're convinced that the world is against them, and they end up being eaten up by negative thoughts, petty jealousies and miseries. They're no fun to be with, they're always complaining and blaming and, not surprisingly, they're nearly always ill.

six exercises to boost your positivity

1 Clasp the fingers of both hands behind your head. Lift your chin and push hard against your hands for 10 seconds. Repeat 5 times.

2 Place your palms against your forehead. Try to push your chin down by pressing your head against your hands. Hold for 10 seconds. Repeat 5 times.

3 Put your left hand against the left side of your head and try to push your left ear towards your left shoulder. At the same time, push your hand against the side of your head. Hold for 10 seconds. Repeat 5 times. Repeat on the right side.

4 Standing or sitting, raise your shoulders as high as you can, with your arms hanging by your sides. Hold for 5 seconds, then let the shoulders drop with their own weight. Repeat 5 times.

5 Standing or sitting, push both shoulders back as far as you can, sticking out your chest and forcing the shoulder blades together. Hold for 5 seconds and relax. Repeat this 3 times.

6 Standing or sitting, push both shoulders as far forward as you can, narrowing the chest and forcing your shoulder blades as far apart as they will go, with your arms hanging down. Hold for 5 seconds and relax. Repeat 3 times.

what to eat for a good night's sleep

Going to bed too full or too hungry both interfere with sleep, as does eating too late, especially if you eat animal protein. This type of food is a mental stimulant and triggers the body to produce more activity hormones. Starchy foods, on the other hand, encourage the body to manufacture more tryptophan – the brain's own calming chemical – as well as the non-active growth and repair hormones. So ideally, evening meals should be based on foods like rice, pasta, potatoes, bread, root vegetables and beans, and you should save the meat meals for the middle of the day.

time for a sandwich

Any sandwich will help, but the best sandwich filling for a good night's sleep is lettuce, a strong soporific. In 1789 one of the great herbalists, Sir John Hill, published his *Family Herbal*. In it he wrote about wild lettuce, used by the ancient Romans as a sleep inducer: 'It eases the most violent pain in colics and other disorders and gently disposes the person to sleep. It has the good effect of a gentle opiate, and none of the bad ones of that violent medicine.' How right he was.

lettuce soup

Perfect as an evening snack as lettuce helps you sleep – and it's a great way to use up a glut of garden lettuces.

4 tbsp extra-virgin olive oil
1 large sweet Spanish onion, very finely chopped
2 cloves garlic, very finely chopped
2 heads Little Gem lettuce, shredded
1 litre vegetable stock
4 large sprigs tarragon, leaves freshly chopped
100ml crème fraîche

Heat the oil and sauté the onion gently for 2 minutes. Add the garlic and continue cooking for a futher minute. Add the shredded lettuce and stir until wilted. Pour in the stock and tarragon and simmer for 5 minutes. Serve with spoonfuls of crème fraîche floating on the top.

pasta with lettuce pesto

A wonderfully healthy pasta dish, providing energy, calcium and protein, plus calming natural chemicals to help you unwind and sleep.

400g fusilli
1 large head radicchio, washed
25g pine kernels
4 tbsp extra-virgin olive oil
4 tbsp Parmesan cheese, freshly grated
1 small handful white lettuce, leaves roughly torn

Cook the pasta in a large saucepan of boiling water according to the packet instructions. Meanwhile, put the radicchio, pine kernels and half the oil into a food processor and whizz until smooth. Keeping the machine running, add the rest of the oil in a gentle stream. When thoroughly blended, pour into a bowl and stir in the cheese and lettuce. Stir the pesto into the pasta and serve.

eat your herbs

Sage, fennel, rosemary and basil are all calming, soothing and sleep-inducing, thanks to the essential oils they contain, so try to include some in your evening meal. Herb teas – especially chamomile and lime blossom – can be as effective as many types of sleeping pills. As well as containing calming chemicals, they are free from caffeine which, for many people, is sleep's greatest enemy.

kids not sleeping?

If your children can't sleep, cut down on their cola intake. Parents would be horrified if someone offered their eight-year-old a double espresso but seem to have no qualms about them getting substantial doses of caffeine from their cola drinks. Is it any wonder that so many youngsters have disturbed sleep patterns, feel tired all day at school, fall behind in their learning and on top of all that develop behavioural difficulties too?

three natural aids to a good night's sleep

1 Extract of passiflora promotes natural sleep. It's perfect if you get to sleep without any problems but keep waking during the night.

2 A standardized extract of valerian calms and soothes away the stresses of a hectic life. It's the answer for people who find it hard getting off to sleep.

3 Lime-blossom tea with added honey helps calm you down before bed.

keep out the light

A good night's sleep is vital, so make sure
your bedroom has curtains which exclude all
light and, if necessary, put lightproof roller
blinds behind them.

check your mattress

In 20 years you may have bought five
toasters, three irons and six cars, yet you may
still be sleeping on the same old mattress.
Once it sags, it won't support you properly
and you won't get the restful, energy-
generating sleep you need.

184

four ways to beat the stress

1 holidays

Taking a long holiday can create almost more stress than staying at work. It requires complex planning and then you may worry while you're away about the work you left behind and the pile that will be waiting for you when you get back. If this happens, it's often more beneficial to take three- or four-day breaks. But don't take your mobile phone and laptop with you, or leave a dozen contact numbers with the people at the office.

2 learn a new skill

Join the local dramatic society, go to painting classes or learn a foreign language. These are great ways of meeting non-work-related people and using a different set of skills.

3 involve the family

If you have a family then involve them in your leisure activities too. It doesn't matter whether it's following a football team, going camping, doing jigsaw puzzles or playing Scrabble together. Activities like these not only represent a huge investment in your physical health, but are an important prop for the emotional health and wellbeing of your entire family unit.

4 make sure you're really having fun

Many people, even when they do make time in their busy schedules for leisure activities, are so afraid that they might be seen to be enjoying themselves that they spend their time doing punishing exercise regimes, obsessional competitive games or 'team-building' activities. This is not leisure for pleasure and does nothing to improve your health. In fact the reverse is true.

ten-point plan for leisure

1 privacy please

Work out a schedule and allocate at least five hours in each working week as private leisure time – and that doesn't include your lunch hour or the time you spend travelling to and from work.

2 weekend leisure

At weekends you must set aside at least one continuous three-hour period or two sets of two hours for leisure activities on your own or with friends and family.

3 relaxation exercises

Use some of your leisure time for relaxation exercises. These will give your mental and emotional energy an immediate boost. Contrary to popular belief, mental therapies like yoga, meditation, visualisation, self-hypnosis and even prayer, are all great stress-busters, which is why they are so effective. Emotional tension creates anxiety, which triggers excessive production of the hormone, adrenaline. This prepares the body for fight or flight, which in turn causes muscle tension. Prolonged periods of this type of stress mean that your muscles are constantly ready for action and permanently in a state of contraction, and this results in pain, discomfort and the relentless burning up of your energy reserves by all that muscular effort.

4 culture vulture

Make sure you channel some of your leisure time into cultural activities. It makes no difference whether these consist of going to pop festivals, discos and clubs, or visiting art galleries, listening to chamber music or going to the opera. It doesn't matter whether you prefer to read sex-and-shopping novels, sci-fi and mysteries, or philosophy, the classics and historical novels. What is important is satisfying your spiritual need for cultural stimulus.

5 playing games

This brings mental energy and is also a brilliant way of building relationships with friends, family and children. You must choose a game that's appropriate to your playing companions, but it doesn't matter whether it's snap or bridge, Monopoly or Scrabble, snakes and ladders or tiddlywinks, charades or Trivial Pursuit. Any of these games will shake up the grey matter and, win or lose, will give you a mental-energy boost. Just keep away from the computer and the Game Boy.

6 get physical

I always have problems when I tell patients who suffer from chronic fatigue that they need to take some physical exercise, as it's the last thing they feel like doing. But getting the body moving releases the feelgood hormones in the brain and the energy-packing activity hormones in the rest of the body. No matter how tired you feel when you get home from work, do something physical.

7 something appropriate

You have to choose a form of activity that is appropriate to your age and general health. If you've been a couch potato for years, don't start with advanced aerobics or long-distance running. Begin slowly and build up to three regular sessions of 20–30 minutes a week. Even a brisk walk – enough to make you sweat and get home slightly out of breath – will start the process off.

8 make it enjoyable

Choose exercise you enjoy – if you hate it you'll never keep it up. Ideally, try to ensure you do a different type of exercise for each period of leisure time that you set aside. Walking, swimming and golf would be a great combination. But you can just as well choose tennis, squash, tenpin-bowling, line dancing, folk dancing, cycling, jogging or even gardening. Just remember that the object is to generate energy, and this will happen automatically the more you exercise.

9 be sensible

If you're getting physical, do take sensible precautions. If you decide to use a mini-scooter, roller blades or a bicycle, then make sure you wear the proper protective gear, as you won't generate much energy lying in a hospital bed with a fractured skull or messed-up kneecap.

10 keep at it

Be committed, be regular and don't allow outside pressures like work to interfere with your leisure time.

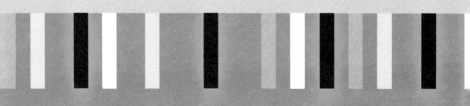

what ever happened to sundays?

78 – the percentage of you who are up and doing by nine o'clock on a Sunday morning, checking your emails, reading your text messages or answering your mobile phone.

50 – the percentage of you who go shopping on a Sunday

25 – the percentage of you who go to work

three worrying things you need to know about shiftwork

1 Driving home after the night shift makes you more likely to have an accident than if you're four times over the alcohol limit.

2 You're 40 per cent more likely to have any sort of an accident, whether it's in the car or at home.

3 Shiftwork kills you early as well as making you tired.

did you know that...?

.... when you should be safely tucked up in bed and sleeping, the body's white-cell count drops so your immune defences are less effective.

...when men have to work late into the night, their jobs may put them at greater risk of physical violence. Late-night petrol-pump attendants and small shop, restaurant or takeaway owners and staff are vulnerable when bars and clubs close.

...if men are on shiftwork, their chances of developing serious heart disease go up by 40 per cent and they're far more likely than other male workers to suffer from lack of energy and chronic fatigue.

...on top of that, shiftworkers commonly suffer from constipation and stomach problems due to dehydration, irregular mealtimes and bad eating habits.

195

196

shortcut to nirvana

• Choose a warm room, turn off the radio or television, disconnect the telephone and lie flat on a very firm bed or on a rug on the floor. Try to empty your mind of all your thoughts and emotions.

• Close your eyes and take three deep, slow breaths in and out.

• Stretch your left leg along the floor away from your body as hard as you can, pointing your foot and contracting the calf, thigh, buttock and lower-back muscles. Hold that position until you feel a slight trembling in the muscles, then relax.

• Repeat with the right leg; then with both legs, and relax again.

• Stretch your left arm down your side, spreading your fingers and pushing from the big muscles at the back of the neck and shoulder so that you contract all the muscles of the upper arm, forearm and hand.

• Relax.

• Repeat with the right arm and relax.

• Repeat with both arms and relax again.

• Stretch both arms and legs together and relax.

• Take five deep breaths and repeat the cycle again. Repeat the cycle four more times.

• Relax totally for 10 minutes, preferably with a blanket within reach, as your body temperature may drop because of your slower heart beat and lower rate of breathing.

meditate on this

Deep meditation can often trigger some unexpected results such as sudden uncontrolled emotional outbursts like laughing or crying. If this happens to you, don't worry. In fact, it's a sign that you really have reached a deep state of relaxation.

• Get into a comfortable position. It doesn't matter if you sit, lie or recline, as long as the radio and television are off, and you've unplugged the telephone.

• Close your eyes.

• Work your way through the Short Cut to Nirvana (pages 196–197).

• Breathe in deeply through your nose and out through your mouth, at the same time trying to empty your mind of all thoughts. While doing this, repeat your chosen mantra – the word 'one' is widely used – preferably out loud and as deeply in your voice register as you can, as this helps to create a vibration.

• Continue breathing deeply and evenly for at least 10 or preferably 20 minutes. Keep pushing away any distracting thoughts while you continue constantly repeating the mantra.

• When you've finished, remain completely still with your eyes closed for 2–3 minutes, then open your eyes but stay where you are for another minute or two.

how stressed are you?

You may not realise how much stress you're under, so how do you tell whether you are suffering from too much? Check the questionnaire below and see how you score. Do you:

• Feel near to tears much of the time?

• Fidget, bite your nails or fiddle with your hair?

• Find it hard to concentrate and impossible to make decisions?

• Find it increasingly hard to talk to people?

• Snap and shout at those around you at home and work?

• Eat when you're not hungry?

• Feel tired much of the time?

• Think that your sense of humour has gone for good?

• Feel suspicious of others?

• No longer have any interest in sex?

• Sleep badly?

• Drink and/or smoke more to help you through those difficult days?

• Ever feel that you just can't cope?

If you answer 'yes' to more than four of these questions, you are stressed. Do something! You can't carry on this way.

de-stress the distress

Here's how to break out of the cycle.

• Do not work more than nine hours a day.

• Take at least half an hour off during the day.

• Take at least one and a half days out of your normal working routine each week.

• Eat regular and healthy meals.

• Take regular exercise.

• Practise some form of relaxation technique.

• Do not use alcohol, caffeine, nicotine, or drugs to relieve stress.

• Remember that stressful situations are not always the unhappy ones.

• Getting married, promoted or moving house all cause stress.

• Learn to recognise your own stress thresholds.

• Use stress positively and channel your energy into making your life better.

blissful massage

A good massage is relaxing, luxurious, pampering and extremely therapeutic. It induces feelings of inner calm, peace and wellbeing, relaxes tense muscles, soothes away headaches and other aches and pains, and relieves physical and emotional tension. And apart from all these wonderful benefits, massage can stimulate the lymph drainage system and speed up the body's elimination processes.

seven massage no-nos

Do not have a massage if you suffer from any of the following:

1 Thrombosis, phlebitis or cellulitis

2 Leg ulcers

3 Inflamed joints after injury or acute arthritis

4 High temperature

5 Varicose veins

6 Unexplained large bruises

7 Any skin condition which is obviously infected, weeping or suppurating.

the four techniques of massage

When giving a massage, use rhythmic, repetitive movements and avoid pressing down on bony areas. Many people like to play their favourite slow music in the background so they can work in time with the rhythm. Western massage is based on four separate techniques that can be used separately or in any combination.

1 Effleurage is a rhythmic, stroking movement that produces physical and mental relaxation. Effleurage movements are always made towards the heart.

2 Petrissage is a bit like kneading bread dough. It's a deep lifting, rolling and squeezing movement, which stimulates muscles and fatty tissue. It's valuable as a way of stretching and relaxing contracted muscles.

3 Applying pressure using small rotating movements of the thumbs, fingertips or heel of the hand. It's used in small specific areas of tension in the neck, shoulders and buttocks. If you're a small person dealing with a large body you can sometimes get more pressure by using the point of your elbow.

4 Percussion is a really hard technique for an amateur to master as it uses fast rhythmic slaps with either a cupped hand or the little finger edge of the hand. It can be used to stimulate skin, blood flow and breathing.

did you know that…?

…the use of essential oils is at least three thousand years old. From the Aztecs to the ancient Greeks and from the Romans to the early Christian Church, the mood-enhancing and medicinal properties of these oils have long been recognised.

four ways to use essential oils

1 You can burn them in a fragrancer so you breathe in their volatile vapours.

2 You can use them as an inhalation. Add three drops to a large bowl of hot water, cover your head and the bowl with a towel, keep your eyes closed and breathe in through the nose and out through the mouth for three or four minutes.

3 You can use them for skin massage. Dilute them with a vegetable carrier oil like grapeseed, sunflower, corn or almond oil and then apply. When making up mixtures for massage oil, don't use more than two drops of essential oil to each large teaspoon of carrier.

4 You can add a few drops to your bathwater, but steer well clear of thyme, basil, clove, cinnamon or peppermint oil as these may irritate the skin. And be sure to avoid direct application of all essential oils during pregnancy without seeking professional advice, as some oils could be harmful.

seven good-mood essential oil mixes

For the massage oils, dilute the total number of drops with one tablespoon of a carrier oil (see page 207).

1 vitality mix

massage – 3 drops lemon, 2 drops geranium, 1 drop frankincense
fragrancer – bergamot
bath – grapefruit

2 brain mix

massage – 2 drops rosemary, 3 drops thyme, 1 drop basil
fragrancer – lemon grass
bath – fennel and juniper

3 snooze mix

massage – 3 drops neroli, 3 drops geranium, 2 drops lavender
fragrancer – lavender
bath – mimosa

4 wake-up mix

massage – 2 drops pine, 4 drops juniper
fragrancer – eucalyptus and lime
bath – juniper

5 sexy mix

massage – 4 drops rose otto, 2 drops jasmine, 2 drops sandalwood
fragrancer – sandalwood
bath – ylang ylang

6 macho mix

massage – 3 drops cedarwood, 2 drops thyme, 2 drops cypress
fragrancer – sandalwood and cinnamon
bath – patchouli

7 sensitive mix

massage – 2 drops jasmine, 2 drops lime blossom, 2 drops neroli, 1 drop carnation
fragrancer – jasmine and carnation
bath – hyacinth

get rid of your anger

Just like excessive stress, anger causes resentment, bitterness and anxiety. Attitudes to letting go of your anger vary enormously. For example, if you're Anglo-Saxon, it's not done to lose your temper, but watch an Italian, Spanish or Greek family eating Sunday lunch and from all the shouting and gesticulating, you'd imagine they were in the middle of a 50-year feud. In reality, they're probably only arguing about whether there's too much salt in the soup.

three ways to let go

1 Physical exercise gets rid of excess energy, encourages self-confidence and offers a safe environment for you to channel your anger in a competitive way. Endurance runners have been shown to be less anxious, more emotionally stable and less prone to irrational outbursts of anger than their physically less active contemporaries.

2 Spend an hour doing your favourite hobby. If sport's not your thing, find out what works for you – maybe gardening or painting, the cinema, theatre or music.

3 Taking your anger out on a punch bag in the bedroom or by hanging a rug in the garden and beating it with a tennis racquet for five minutes are both great ways of dealing with a frustrating day when the boss has been on your back or you've been given a parking ticket.

two things you didn't know about smiling

1 It requires much more effort to frown than to smile as frowning uses many more of your facial muscles.

2 Smiling brings skin-protective benefits. There's now a mass of scientific evidence proving conclusively that positive attitudes enhance the body's immune defences and so protect your skin – and all your other organs too – from the ageing damage of free radicals.

did you know that…?

…colour has been used as a mood-enhancing and therapeutic tool for at least two thousand years. Shamans, mystics, the physicians of ancient Greece, priests of almost every known religion, the great architects and artists of history and the psychiatrists of our modern age – all have discovered the immense power of colour.

did you know that…?

… wearing black, grey or beige clothes can feed negative emotions such as sadness and depression? And once you're feeling down, you'll inevitably choose these colours, which means you're trapped in a downward spiral.

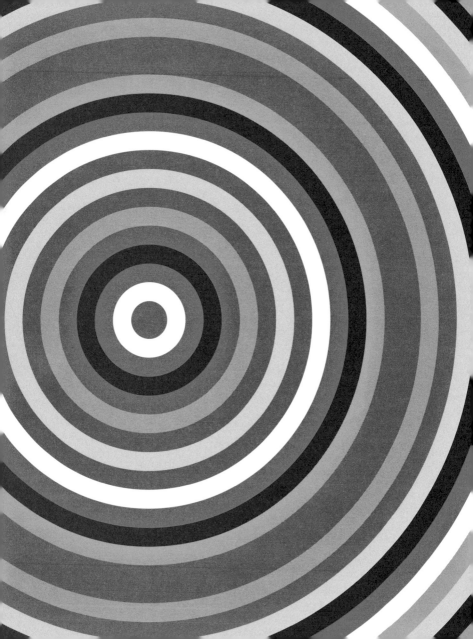

looking
good

four reasons why home-made is best for skin, hands, nails and hair

1 What you make at home is incredibly cheap. You're not paying for the advertising or the environmentally damaging packaging.

2 You avoid the damaging chemical additives that are used in the vast majority of commercially available products.

3 Most importantly, home-made products work better than most products that you buy over the counter.

4 You avoid exposure to chemicals which, if you use them during pregnancy, can have a damaging effect on the fertility of boys.

made in a minute

- a jug of chamomile tea as a hair rinse
- a bowl of warm olive oil to nourish the finger nails
- rosewater and glycerin for beautiful smooth hands
- lemon juice to clean and whiten cuticles
- garlic and vinegar to cure fungal infections

live yoghurt and salt scrub

Simply add 2 teaspoons coarse sea salt to a carton of yoghurt, spread it evenly over your face and leave for 10 minutes. Then, using cold water, gently rub the mixture all over the skin until it's rinsed off completely.

The salt acts as a gentle exfoliator and antiseptic and the natural bacteria in the yoghurt provide a protective layer that will fight off any other bugs and so help to prevent the formation of spots. Do this at least twice a week.

bath-time oats for inflamed skin

Put 4 tablespoons uncooked oats in a muslin bag, hang the bag under the tap as you run the bath, then use the bag to clean your skin. The natural oils and vitamins in the oats will soothe inflamed areas and stimulate the growth of new skin. Use for three or four baths before replacing the oats.

avocado aware

Avocados are nature's gift to the skin. They are not only wonderfully nutritious but avocado oil makes a great skin food. After you've eaten your avocado, rub your skin with the inside of the peel and massage in the oily film that's left behind.

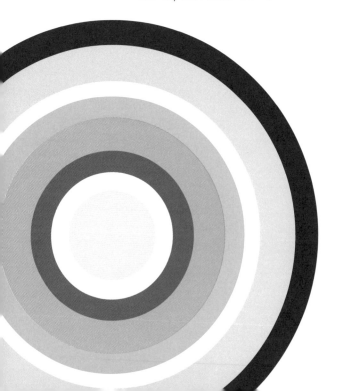

chilled avocado soup

This gives you the legendary skin benefits of avocados, which are rich in vitamin E and antioxidants. Add to that the circulation-boosting properties of chilli and cayenne pepper, the protective bacteria in the yoghurt and lots of zinc from the pumpkin seeds.

5 ripe avocados
1 litre vegetable stock
juice of 1 lemon
2 large cloves garlic,
  finely chopped
2 red chillies, deseeded
  and chopped
$1/2$ tbsp cayenne
  pepper
5 spring onions,
  roughly chopped
1 x 200g can tomatoes
150g live natural
  yoghurt
25g pumpkin seeds

Put the avocado flesh into a food processor or large blender with the next 7 ingredients and whizz until smooth. Add the yoghurt and whizz again for a few seconds. Spoon into a bowl and leave to cool in the fridge. Dry-fry the pumpkin seeds in a small frying pan. Remove the pan from the heat and leave to cool. Sprinkle the pumpkin seeds on the soup just before serving.

orange face mask

Purée the flesh of a whole orange, spread
it over your face, leave for 20 minutes, then
rinse off with tepid water. This leaves the skin
feeling clean and stimulated. Your skin will
also have absorbed some of the orange's
vitamin C, betacarotene and a complex of
bioflavonoids called vitamin P which
strengthen the tiny capillaries, so protecting
you from unsightly broken veins.

more food and face mask treats

- Honey

- Carrot grated into olive oil

- Grape juice (or peeled and crushed fresh grapes)

cinnamon toast with figs

What a wonderful start to a leisurely day – and a great skin boost too! The eggs in this delicious recipe contain iron, B vitamins and protein and there are cleansing essential oils in the cumin. Added to this, there's the ultimate pleasure of combining those delicious flavours with fresh figs, known since ancient times as one of nature's great skin foods.

4 eggs
2 tsp ground cinnamon
4 medium slices
   wholemeal bread
75g butter
2 tbsp dark brown
   sugar
4 fresh figs, halved
   lengthways, to serve

Beat the eggs with half the cinnamon in a large bowl. Slice the bread into thick fingers. Melt the butter in a frying pan. Dip the bread in the egg mixture and fry in the butter on both sides until golden. Sprinkle with the brown sugar and extra cinnamon. Serve with the figs on the side.

lavender tonic

Lavender has been known for years to do wonders for the skin. Steep the tops of fresh lavender sprigs in white wine vinegar for a week (shake the bottle occasionally), then dilute 1 part of the vinegar to 4 parts water and use as a skin tonic.

oil-purpose

Almond oil is used as a base for many natural skin products. You can make your own oil treatments by adding a couple of drops of your favourite essential oil to one tablespoon almond oil. For oily skin, use chamomile, lavender or rose essential oils, while neroli or clary sage are good for older skins. Spread the oil mixture on your face and leave for 20 minutes before washing off and applying a skin tonic.

stir-fried turkey breast with vegetables and noodles

Turkey mixed with skin-nourishing root vegetables and circulation-stimulating ginger and chilli makes an all-year-round skin-enhancing recipe.

400g egg noodles
2 tbsp rapeseed oil
2.5cm fresh root ginger, grated
10 cloves garlic, peeled
1 red chilli, deseeded and finely chopped
450g turkey breast, finely cubed
1 small onion, finely chopped
450g finely chopped mixed vegetables (baby carrots, broccoli, mangetout, sweetcorn, cauliflower, cabbage, or a packet of stir-fry vegetables)
2 tbsp sesame oil
1 tbsp soy sauce

Cook the noodles according to the packet instructions. Meanwhile, heat the oil in a preheated wok or large saucepan and stir-fry the ginger, garlic, chilli and turkey for 2 minutes. Add the onion and vegetables and stir in the sesame oil. Stir-fry for a further 4 minutes, adding the soy sauce gradually, until the vegetables are just beginning to crisp. Remove from the heat. Drain the cooked noodles, mix into the stir-fry and serve immediately.

facial sauna

Use fresh herbs for a facial sauna. Put a handful into a pan, pour boiling water over, cover the pan, leave to infuse for 10 minutes, then reheat. Remove from the heat, transfer to a heatproof bowl and lean over the steaming bowl with a towel over your head.

- **Lavender** to heal and soothe the skin

- **Rosemary** to heal and stimulate the circulation

- **Marigold** to heal

- **Cornflower** to refresh

- **Mallow**, **marigold** and **sage** for problem skins

- **Comfrey** and **borage flowers** for dry skin

- **Thyme** to open your pores and get your blood really pumping

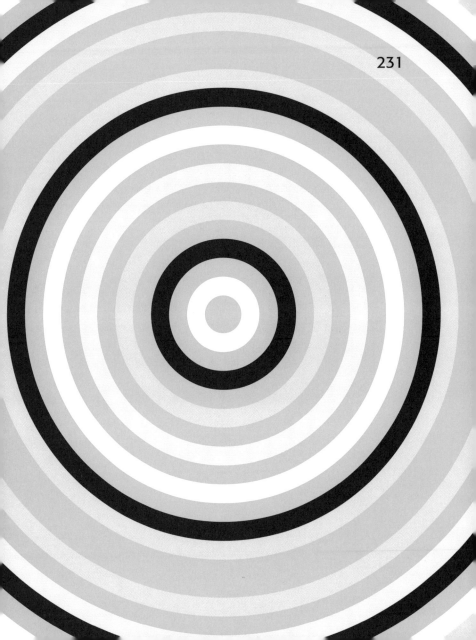

the magic of tea tree oil

Although the Aborigines have used tea tree oil for centuries as a treatment for cuts and wounds, it wasn't studied scientifically until the 1920s and it took another 70 years for its antiseptic and antibiotic properties to be accepted.

Use it for spots, infected nails, cold sores, dandruff, coughs, sinus problems, sore throats and other infections. Studies published by Middlesex University in London show that tea tree oil is even effective against life-threatening antibiotic-resistant bacteria.

salad vegeçoise

Radiance on a plate, thanks to the skin-nourishing betacarotene in the peppers, the B vitamins in the eggs and all the natural oils in the olives.

1 large Iceberg lettuce, roughly shredded
$1/2$ cucumber, peeled, deseeded and sliced
1 red pepper, deseeded and cubed
6 tomatoes, quartered and deseeded
4 eggs, hardboiled and quartered
12 black olives, stoned
100ml home-made vinaigrette

Put the lettuce into a large, wide bowl. Arrange the other salad vegetables on top. Place the eggs and olives around the side of the bowl. Pour the dressing over the salad and serve.

twelve kitchen remedies
for hair

jojoba oil

1

This conditions and adds lustre to the hair.
Heat a couple of tablespoons of jojoba oil, apply
it to the roots, then comb it through the hair.
Wrap a warm towel around your head and leave
it for 30 minutes, then use a very mild shampoo
to wash the oil out.

2 ginger root with sesame oil

Together these make a very stimulating hair conditioner. Squeeze the juice of the fresh ginger root into a couple of tablespoons of sesame oil, apply to the hair and wrap your head in a warm towel. Leave it on for as long as possible before shampooing.

3 rosemary

Traditionally used to stimulate blood circulation.
Add a handful to cold water, simmer for
15 minutes, then swab the roots of your hair
with the mixture before shampooing.

Nettles are rich in the minerals needed for healthy hair growth. Try to wash your hair daily in a mild non-detergent nettle shampoo. Steam young nettletops to eat with a knob of butter and a little nutmeg, then use the steaming water to rub into your scalp.

4
nettles

5 onion

This is a wonderful source of sulphur, which is essential for healthy hair. As well as including onions in your diet, rubbing raw onion over the roots of your hair before you shampoo will stimulate your scalp.

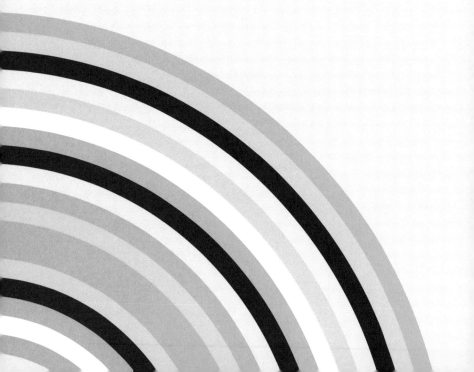

Use a chamomile shampoo and add a cup of cider vinegar to 500ml hot water for the final rinse. In addition, massage your scalp thoroughly at bedtime with witch hazel extract or add a few drops of tea tree oil to your normal shampoo.

You can also make a final rinse from a dozen or so globe artichoke leaves, simmered for 10 minutes, then strained and cooled. Alternatively, use catmint tea – a generous handful of chopped catmint leaves steeped in boiling water for 10 minutes, strained and left to cool.

6

for dandruff

for 7 fair hair

To enhance blonde hair, make a final rinse from an infusion of mullein, strained and cooled, or from chamomile or from a nettle teabag.

8 for dark hair

Condition with a solution of 1 cup beetroot juice to 4 cups hot water mixed with a teaspoon of salt. Massage through the hair, then rinse out.

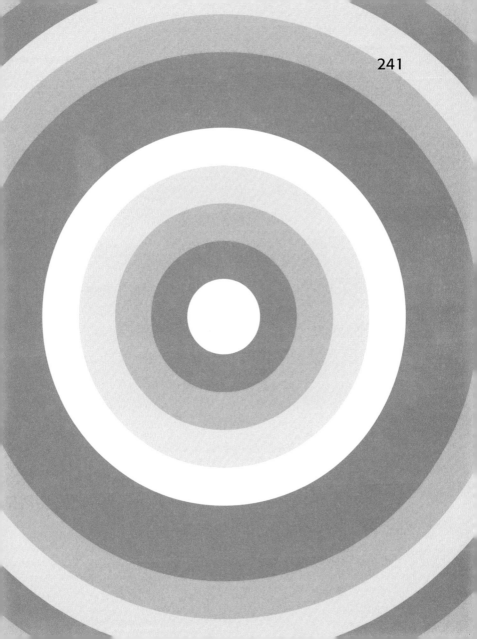

9 to cover grey

Avoid horrible commercial dyes yet cover your grey by using sage. Add 4 tablespoons of chopped leaves to a jug of boiling water, cover and leave for at least half an hour before straining. Use a brush or sponge to apply the liquid to the grey roots. Don't wash out.

10

To make the ideal shampoo for oily hair, mix together half a cup of rosewater, two whole eggs and a generous dash of dark rum.

for oily hair

Warm a cup of olive oil in a bowl of hot water, massage it into the scalp and hair, wrap your head in a towel for an hour, then shampoo and rinse with the chamomile and cider-vinegar mix (see page 239).

11

for dry hair

for dry hair

12

Add an egg yolk and a teaspoon of natural gelatin dissolved in a little boiling water to your favourite herbal shampoo.

sweetcorn and haddock chowder

Haddock is a rich source of iodine, lack of which can lead to dry, lifeless hair, coarseness of the skin and chronic exhaustion. Iodine is also essential for the normal function of the thyroid gland, which controls the body's metabolism.

350g smoked haddock
700ml semi-skimmed milk
2 bay leaves
50g unsalted butter
1 large onion, very finely chopped
1 clove garlic, very finely chopped
225g potatoes, peeled and finely cubed
200g sweetcorn, frozen or canned
300ml single cream

Poach the haddock in the milk with the bay leaves for about 5 minutes. Remove the bay leaves and discard. Remove the fish with a slotted spoon and flake the flesh with a fork. Reserve the poaching liquid. Heat the butter in a saucepan and sauté the onion and garlic gently until soft. Add the potatoes and the reserved poaching liquid and simmer until tender. Add the sweetcorn, then stir in the fish and cream and heat through for 5 minutes or until the sweetcorn is tender. Serve immediately.

did you know that...?

...contrary to popular belief, nails aren't made of calcium but of a horny material called keratin, and they grow from the root end at a speed of roughly one millimetre a week.

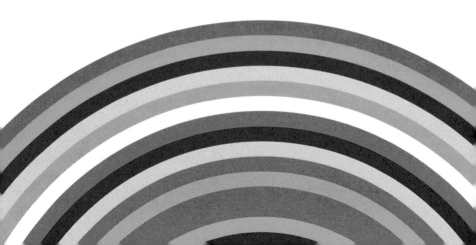

supplements for healthy nails

• To encourage strong nails and healthy growth, you need complex B vitamins, zinc and pantothenic acid – remember, there's a rich supply of pantothenic acid in avocados – together, of course, with a generally sensible and healthy diet.

• Most people think that white spots on the nails are a sign of calcium deficiency, but in fact they're nearly always caused by a lack of zinc. Eat a handful of pumpkin seeds every day to get your supply. Shellfish are another enormously rich source of zinc and, best of all, are oysters, as long as you're not allergic to them.

• One of the traditional foods for healthy nails is gelatin, which you can now get as a special nail-formula capsule.

• Last but not least, eat garlic. This amazing little bulb has powerful anti-fungal properties – perfect for those unsightly fungal nail infections.

fungal nail infections

Bathe the affected nails in a mixture of 250ml warm water, 15ml cider vinegar and two crushed cloves of garlic. This will help athlete's foot as well.

brittle nails

Make sure you eat 10ml extra-virgin olive oil each day and soak your nails once a week in a bowl of warm olive oil. After 10 minutes, wipe off the surplus. You can also strengthen your nails by soaking them in an infusion of dried horsetail.

reddened or chafed hands

Make a soft paste of ground almonds and a little rosewater and spread it on your hands like a face mask. Leave on for about half an hour, then wipe off the surplus.

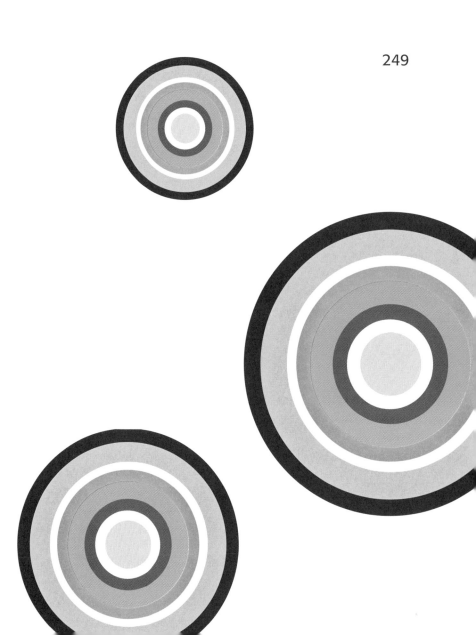

two bedtime treats for hands

1 Mix together equal parts of rosewater and glycerin and rub into your hands at bedtime. You can wear soft cotton gloves during the night to boost the effect.

2 In a small bottle, mix 50ml almond oil with 25 drops chamomile, lavender or benzoin essential oil and add a vitamin E capsule. Warm the bottle under a hot tap, then at bedtime, just massage the mixture into your hands. Sleep tight!

the best home-made barrier cream

Mix together 5g kaolin (stocked by most pharmacies), 5g cold-pressed almond oil and the yolk of one large organic egg. Rub the mixture well into the hands, particularly around the cuticles and under the nails before you start your work. When you've finished your dirty tasks, simply scrub off with a soft bristle brush, leaving the hands clean and the skin soft and undamaged.

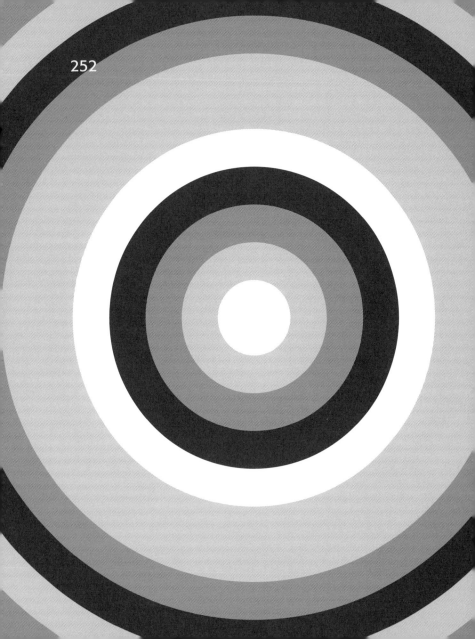

252

lemons for hands

Always have fresh lemons in your kitchen.
The flesh and juice rubbed into your hands
not only help keep your hands clean but
they whiten the skin, are strongly antiseptic
and are an effective deodorant if you've been
handling onions, garlic or fish.

oats for hands

There are plenty of oat-based commercial
products for hand and skin care on the
market, but save your money. Simply take
a scoop of oats out of your porridge packet,
put them in your cupped hand, add some
water and rub your hands together until the
oats form a paste. Massage this thoroughly in
every nook and cranny of your hands, fingers,
cuticles and nails, then rinse off. The fibre is
an effective cleanser, but you'll also absorb
vitamin E and other radiance-boosting
nutrients through the skin.

chocolate for hands

Sorry, you don't get to eat it! But if you've had a heavy session in the garden, been redecorating the house, or your job involves working with tools so you end up with calloused, hard hands, mix cocoa butter, beeswax and cold-pressed almond oil in equal proportions and warm them very slowly in a heatproof bowl over a saucepan of boiling water. When they're all blended together, remove from the heat and keep stirring until the mixture sets. Keep in a jam jar wrapped in foil and use as hand cream every night.

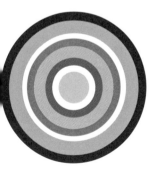
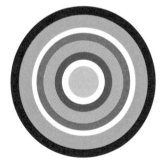

pineapple for hands

Fresh pineapple contains the enzyme bromelaine which is a highly effective digestive enzyme that also softens the cuticles. Make a large glass of fresh pineapple juice, put 30ml into a jug with 3ml cider vinegar and 5ml extra-virgin olive oil. Whisk together and soak your nails in it for at least 15 minutes. Drink the rest of the juice!

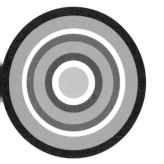
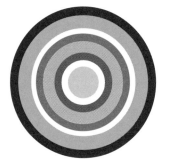
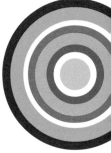

did you know that…?

…we are all born with good posture.
You only have to look at the way babies
hold themselves when they first start to sit,
crawl and walk. Their bodies achieve good
posture naturally and with the minimum
amount of effort. Unfortunately, though,
learned behaviour soon takes over and
thanks to badly designed furniture, acquired
habits, sitting all day at a computer, lack
of exercise and general laziness, our bodies
suffer from chronic misalignment and we
need a much greater muscular effort to
hold ourselves up. This results in muscular
tension and physical problems like head,
neck, shoulder and low-back pain, and
often breathing and digestive difficulties
too. Every movement we make drains our
energy resources. No wonder we feel tired!

how a glass of water and a straw can be good for your face

These exercises were developed to help people who had suffered strokes and other neurological problems, but they have cosmetic benefits too as they build tone in your facial muscles. They also stimulate the blood flow to the cells of the skin and to the skin's nerve supply.

Repeat each exercise three times and try to repeat them all at least three times a week. Do them in front of your partner, children or grandchildren and everyone will have a good laugh as well and, as you know, laughter is the best medicine.

All you need are a large glass of water and a packet of thick plastic straws.

• With a straw in the middle of your lips and the other end under the water, breathe in through your nose and very slowly out through the straw to produce a constant stream of bubbles.

• Repeat as above, but with the straw in the left-hand corner of your mouth.

• Repeat as above, but in the right-hand corner of your mouth.

• Suck a mouthful of water through the straw as quickly as you can and swallow.

• Suck a mouthful of water as slowly as you can and swallow.

• Suck a mouthful of water and blow it back into the glass as quickly as you can.

• Suck a mouthful of water and blow it back into the glass as slowly as you can.

• Blow air through the straw into the water as hard as you can with your cheeks held in.

• Blow air through the straw into the water as hard as you can with your cheeks puffed out.

• Do this exercise in front of a mirror – raise your left eyebrow, raise your right eyebrow, purse your lips, blow a raspberry, suck in your cheeks, blow out your cheeks, blow another raspberry.

non-meatballs in tomato sauce

There's a double radiance bonus in this dish, which comes from the radiant-friendly nutrients in the vegeburger mix and also from the lycopene in the tomatoes. Lycopene is one of the most powerful natural protective antioxidants. It also stimulates new skin cell growth, slows the skin's ageing process and is a mighty wrinkle-zapper.

450g vegeburger mix
3 cloves garlic, finely
  chopped
2 tbsp mint, freshly
  chopped leaves
2 tbsp parsley, freshly
  chopped leaves
1 x 400g can tomatoes
1 vegetable stock cube
4 tbsp white wine
1 large onion, finely
  chopped
1 tbsp extra-virgin
  olive oil
1 green chilli,
  deseeded and finely
  chopped
100ml rapeseed oil

Prepare the vegeburger mix according to the packet instructions, adding the garlic, mint and parsley. Put the tomatoes and their juice into a large frying pan with the crumbled stock cube, wine, onion, olive oil and chilli. Bring to the boil and simmer for 10 minutes. While the sauce is cooking, form the vegeburger mixture into walnut-sized balls and fry gently in the rapeseed oil for 3 minutes on each side. Add them to the tomato sauce and serve immediately.

fresh cherry tarts

As well as skin-nourishing protective antioxidants and masses of vitamin C, cherries contain substantial quantities of bio-flavonoids, which slow down the skin's ageing process.

1 sheet ready-made
  puff pastry
450g fresh cherries,
  stoned
2 eggs
250g live natural
  yoghurt
2 tbsp caster sugar
2 tbsp cherry brandy

Preheat the oven to 220°C/425°F/Gas 7. Grease 4 individual loose-bottomed tart tins, roll out the pastry, divide into 4 and use to line the tart tins. Put the cherries on top of the pastry. Beat the eggs together in a bowl. Put the yoghurt, half the sugar and the cherry brandy into a bowl and beat in the eggs. Pour the mixture into the tins, scatter the remaining sugar on top and bake in the preheated oven for 25 minutes, or until the filling has risen and turned a golden colour.

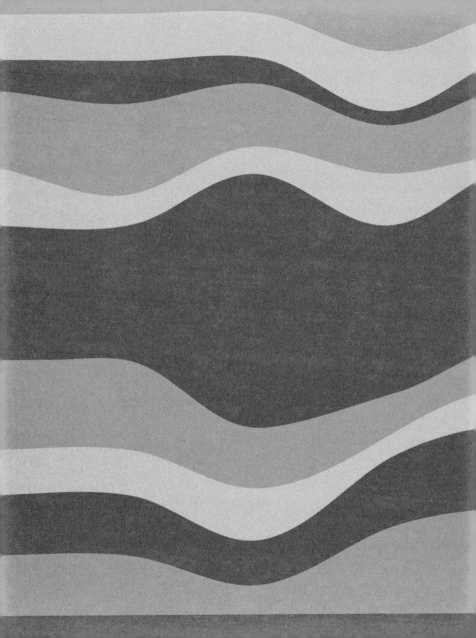

at home and work

try these for a healthy home

• Clear the clutter – there is nothing so fatiguing as living in a constant muddle. Fight against the magpie instinct and stop being a hoarder.

• Get rid of stuff you don't need.

• Make sure your home is well ventilated and turn the heating down a couple of degrees.

• More fresh air and a cooler temperature help generate more physical energy.

• Think about redecorating. Drab colours make for drab people – beige is enervating. You don't have to use crimson and gold, but lively colours generate their own energy.

• Check all heating appliances annually as even low levels of carbon monoxide from unserviced heaters are a common cause of chronic fatigue and high levels could be fatal.

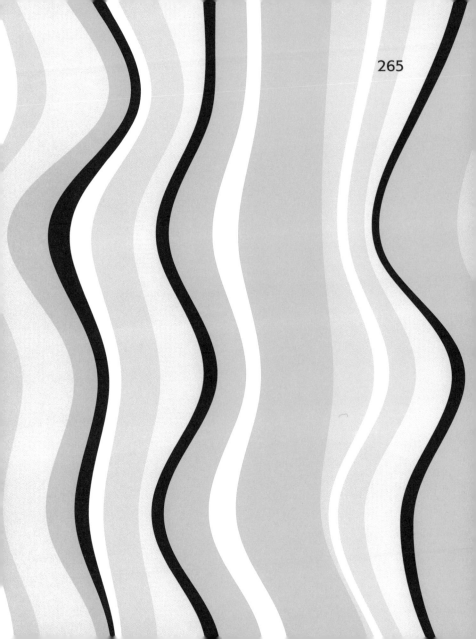

five minutes to freshness

• Fresh flowers in the house are great givers of energy – a vase of daffodils in the spring, wild hedgerow flowers in the summer, a few twigs of autumn leaves or a bowl of scented hyacinths at Christmas are all signs of Nature's vigour that you can enjoy in your home.

• Bring fragrance into your home with real herbal pot pourri, and banish forever artificially scented air fresheners, fake aromatherapy candles and room deodorisers. The synthetic musk perfumes they contain are all toxic and de-energising.

two ways to wash away your troubles

1 Turn your bathroom into a spa by adding invigorating essential oils like rosemary, pine or eucalyptus to your bath.

2 Take a cold bath or shower. These are very stimulating and push the body into producing extra energy. When you've finished washing, slowly add cold water to the bath while rubbing your arms, legs and stomach briskly with a rough flannel or loofah. If you're having a shower, turn the temperature down gradually. Once the water is really cold, stay in it for at least 10 seconds, then dry yourself as briskly as possible with a rough towel. You may think it sounds awful, but once you've tried it you'll be hooked.

ten-point plan to maximise your energy at work

1 Start your day with a good breakfast to maximise your energy potential (see pages 64–71).

2 Drink at least one and a half litres of water between arriving at work and going home to combat the effects of air conditioning and central heating in the workplace. You'll feel more comfortable generally and will be less at risk of getting headaches.

3 Surround your own workspace with loads of green plants, particularly ivies and spider plants. Plants not only give off moisture, which increases humidity and makes the atmosphere more comfortable, but they absorb pollutants from electronic machinery such as computers and printers.

4 Increase your energy levels by always switching off electrical appliances when they're not being used. If you leave them in standby mode, they still produce ozone.

5 If you're using a computer for long periods, set a kitchen timer for 30 minutes. When it pings, sit back in your chair, look out of the window or across the room, and give your eyes and brain a 2-minute break. In addition, make sure you look away from the screen for at least 30 seconds every 15 minutes and focus your eyes on a distant object.

6 If you frequently use a keyboard and the telephone at the same time, you must have a hands-free headset. Keeping the telephone wedged between your ear and shoulder guarantees headaches, stiff necks, painful shoulders, backache and constant fatigue.

7 Organise your desk or workstation to suit you. It's no good having the telephone on the right-hand side if you're left-handed. Have an ergonomic chair that is fully adjustable to suit your size and shape and have a footstool too. This will maximise your comfort, minimise muscular effort and conserve your much-needed energy.

8 Use your lunch break to re-charge your energy. Don't sit at your desk with a sandwich but get out of the office, even if it's raining. A short walk stimulates your circulation and breathing, which increases oxygen levels and stimulates your metabolism to produce more energy.

9 Eat to beat office pollution. Have a generous portion of at least two of the following foods every day: carrots, red or yellow peppers, apricots, strawberries, blackberries, blueberries, spinach, watercress, spring greens, broccoli, sweet potatoes, cantaloupe melon, tomatoes, and dark green or red lettuce.

10 Get into the habit of standing up during telephone calls. Shift your weight from foot to foot, do some gentle knee bends, take a few steps each way, stand on tiptoe a few times – all of this works the muscle pump in your calves and stimulates better blood flow.

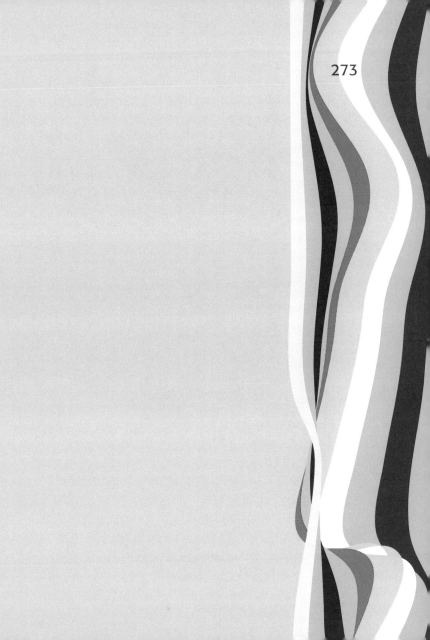

catnap

A 10-minute catnap can restore your physical activity levels, or a few minutes spent in simple meditation can stimulate an immediate increase in your mental energy.

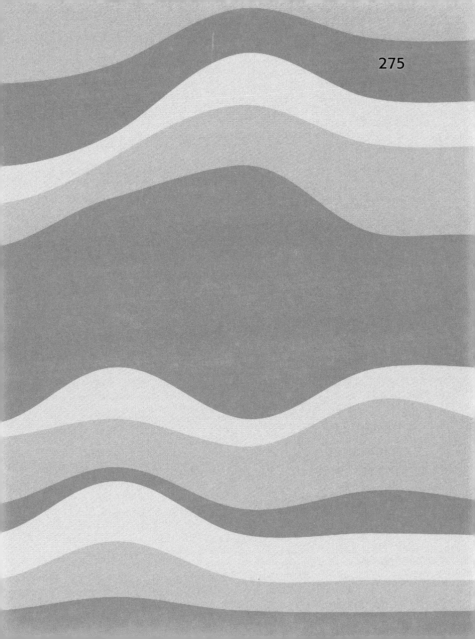

workplace eats

• Always carry a bag of mixed dried fruits, nuts and seeds. They'll give you a balance of instant and slow-release energy, plus masses of vitamins and minerals.

• Eat as wide a variety of foods as you can. If you always eat the same lunchtime sandwich or soup, or take the same potato to pop in the workplace microwave, you don't get the spread of essential nutrients that you need.

• When winter comes, take a couple of wholemeal rolls and a thermos of high-energy hot food to work – a home-made vegetable soup or a warming casserole or stew. Also take some fresh fruit and you've got an energy-giving, sustaining and nourishing feast.

• Try not to eat at your desk or workstation. If there's a works canteen, there must be something healthy on the menu. If not, go out for the occasional pizza and salad or for a takeaway shish kebab in pitta bread.

• Pitta bread and raw vegetable sticks with a pot of hummus, guacamole or taramosalata, and a piece of exotic fresh fruit like kiwi, paw-paw or mango make an interesting energy-boosting lunchtime variation.

hummus

One of the best – and simplest – things you can eat for lunch at work, and easy to pack. Try it with pitta bread or raw vegetables and follow with fruit. Worktime energy on a plate!

1 x 400g can
   chickpeas, drained
   and washed
juice of 1 lemon
2 cloves garlic, peeled
   and finely grated
3 large sprigs mint,
   roughly torn, and 4
   sprigs left whole
2 tbsp extra-virgin
   olive oil

Put the first 3 ingredients and the torn mint into a blender or food processor and whizz until blended. Keep the machine running and gradually add the olive oil until the mixture is smooth. Transfer to a serving dish. Garnish with mint sprigs and serve.

leek and potato soup

This soup is a great source of energy, so take it to work for lunch, eat it hot or cold, and amaze your colleagues with your afternoon energy levels.

4 tbsp extra-virgin olive oil
2 large leeks, trimmed and roughly chopped
450g potatoes, peeled and cubed
1.2 litres chicken stock
4 tbsp flat-leaf parsley, finely chopped leaves, plus extra to garnish
500g live natural yoghurt

Heat the oil in a large saucepan and sauté the leeks gently for about 10 minutes. Add the potatoes and continue to cook for about 5 minutes. Pour in the stock and simmer until the potatoes are tender, about 15 minutes. Transfer to a blender or food processor and whizz until smooth. Return to the heat, add the parsley and simmer for 5 minutes. Stir in the yoghurt and garnish with the extra parsley. For a cold version, strain the mixture after it has been whizzed. Mix in the yoghurt, but omit the chopped parsley and garnish with chopped leaves.

colour at work

• Industrial psychologists advise companies on the best colours to use in offices, factories and workshops in order to enhance the work people do. The colour you wear affects the way you perform too.

• If you're going to a meeting which you know will be stressful, women can try wearing a pale blue scarf or men a pale blue pocket handkerchief. This calming and soothing colour will help keep both your and your colleagues' stress levels down.

• For complex financial negotiations, when you know you'll need to concentrate hard, add some yellow – men can wear yellow braces, women yellow shoes or a yellow handbag.

• And if you know you're in for a very long and boring conference programme, wear red. This stimulating colour will help keep you and those around you awake, and you'll still be looking good at the end of the day.

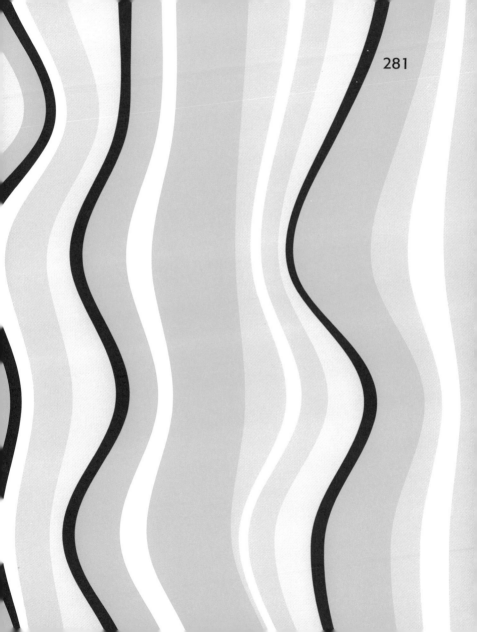

colour at home

People used to paint the rooms of their house in different colours according to the activities that went on there – reds for dining rooms to stimulate conversation and the intellect, greens for the library to aid concentration and calm when reading, the palest yellows for the most restful bedrooms, and terracotta and pinks for elegant, restrained sitting rooms. Why not take a tip from the past and try it yourself?

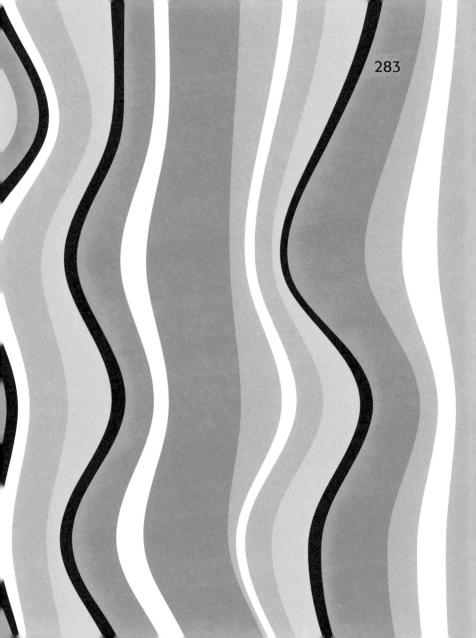

283

is your washing-up liquid making you ill?

Most washing-up liquids contain synthetic musk fragrances which are persistent and toxic chemicals. Residues can be left on cutlery and crockery that is not well rinsed, and these residues will then contaminate food. They can also be absorbed through the skin and, because they dissolve in fat, they end up as long-term deposits in the body, posing a threat to all of us but especially to small children. Look out for 'green' versions and the better supermarket own-label products. The good ones will list all the ingredients; the risky ones won't.

is your antibacterial surface cleaner making you ill?

These too contain hazardous synthetic musks (see page 285) but consumers are brainwashed to believe these cleaners are necessary to kill every known bug. However, there is growing evidence that this obsession with over-zealous hygiene is one probable cause of the ever-increasing amount of childhood allergies. So when you need to disinfect a surface, buy one of the environmentally safer products or save your money and simply use vinegar and hot water.

is your oven cleaner making you ill?

Oven cleaners are likely to contain highly toxic chemicals called phthalates as well as synthetic musks (see page 285). 'Green' versions are available, but they may need a bit more elbow-grease.

are your laundry products making you ill?

Fabric softeners and other laundry products also often contain synthetic musks (see page 285), which are now so widespread that they can be found in almost everyone's body fat – and women accumulate twice as much as men. Synthetic musks even turn up in breast milk so are a serious danger to your baby. 'Green' alternatives are widely available.

are the plastics around your house making you ill?

• Plastics are a major hazard to babies and small children. Vinyl flooring is made from PVC and, to keep it pliable, it contains plasticisers called phthalates. These interfere with our hormones and have been blamed for early puberty, birth defects, damage to testicles and infertility. Some plasticisers have already been banned from teething rings and soft toys for small children.

• Replace vinyl with linoleum which is non-toxic and has natural antiseptic properties. Slate, quarry tiles or natural wood are also ideal alternatives, as is natural cork flooring. It's warmer and 100 per cent non-toxic.

• Polystyrene food containers are also made with chemicals that are believed to affect human oestrogens. And to prevent toxic substances getting into food, avoid direct contact with plastic film by keeping food in glass or ceramic containers with the film stretched over the top.

are the descalers and air fresheners you use making you ill?

Most toilet descalers contain synthetic musks (see page 285) as do air fresheners. The most dangerous of these is xylene, which is known to cause cancer in animals. Lavatory bleaches are one of the worst culprits. Apart from being extremely poisonous, nearly all contain highly toxic chlorine. This converts to organochlorines which persist in the environment and are stored in body tissues. As a safe and environmentally friendly alternative, use baking soda or white vinegar and leave them in the toilet overnight.

is the soap you wash with making you ill?

When you're out shopping for soap, stick to the natural, eco-friendly sort. They're better for your skin too.

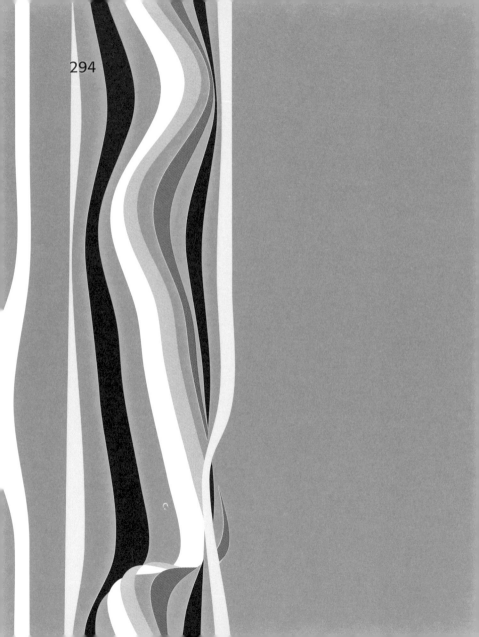
294

is your carpet making you ill?

Your carpet could well contain adhesives which release volatile organic compounds (VOCs) into the air. A carpet also plays host to a wealth of chemicals designed to resist stains, repel moths, kill dustmites and prevent static, but which are all potentially damaging to humans. Samples taken from carpets have also been found to contain tributyl tin (TBT), one of the most potent endocrine-disrupting chemicals there is and a cause of sexual mutation in animals.

On top of this, insecticides, pesticides, solvents, air fresheners, lead, mercury, dustmite droppings and a host of other damaging substances are found in carpet dust. These can affect children and adults and are a common cause of asthma. Wooden flooring is an alternative but avoid laminates as these use toxic adhesives. Sisal, coir and seagrass are other alternatives and are mostly grown without the use of chemicals.

is your furniture polish making you ill?

Before using polish, take care, as most manufacturers will not disclose the chemicals they use and I can only assume they must be nasty, otherwise they'd come clean. Traditional beeswax may be harder work, but it won't release VOCs into the air at home for your family to inhale.

dustmites and tiny tots

Avoid anti-dustmite insecticides, especially in a child's room. They are a permanent risk and can be inhaled or get onto the skin.

the lead effect

Lead is one of the most dangerous substances, especially because it is has a cumulative effect. Modern paints don't contain lead but watch out for old paints. If you live in an old house, get professional advice before redecorating. Never rub down old lead-based paint or use a blowtorch on it, nor burn old windows, doors or other painted timber. And watch out for the fact that many older houses may still contain sections of lead piping in their water system. If you're worried, contact your water supplier.

solvent story

Paints, stains, varnishes and wood preservatives – even some water-based versions – also contain solvents, which can be just as worrying as lead (see opposite). These can affect blood cells, and may trigger asthma, headaches and migraine. And, like all volatile organic compounds (VOCs), they contribute to summer smog. There are lots of natural alternatives to choose from on the market.

an organic outdoors

If there's one place that must be organic it should be your garden. Garden chemicals damage the immune system and are a common cause of accidental poisoning in children. Use a natural alternative. Remember, too, that exterior timber is mostly treated with arsenic compounds which leach into soil leaving a highly toxic residue. This gets into grass and plants, and is brought into the house on human and animal feet, adding to the toxic chemical load deposited forever in your flooring. Again, there are alternative timber treatments, so ask before buying fencing, decking and play equipment.

no smoke without fire

The autumn garden bonfire may give off frightening amounts of poisonous smoke, as may the cosy wood fire in your grate.

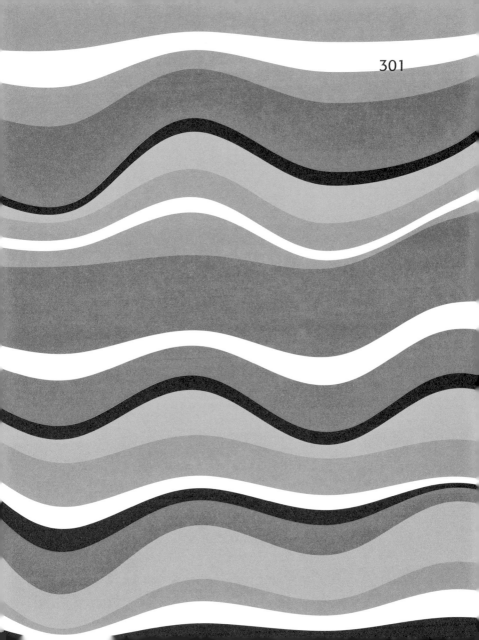

index

Editorial Director Jane O'Shea
Art Director Helen Lewis
Designer Claire Peters
Project Editor Hilary Mandleberg
Production Ruth Deary
Recipes Sally van Straten

This edition first published in 2006
by Quadrille Publishing Limited
Alhambra House
27–31 Charing Cross Road
London WC2H OLS

Reprinted in 2006
10 9 8 7 6 5 4 3 2

The rights of Michael van Straten
and Sally Pearce to be identified as
the authors of this work have been
asserted by them in accordance
with the Copyright, Design and
Patents Act 1988.

British Library Cataloguing-in-
Publication Data
A catalogue record for this book is
available from the British Library.

ISBN-13: 978 184400 269 6
ISBN-10: 1 84400 269 1

Printed in Singapore

Answers for page 167:
1 112
2 11
3 48
4 6
5 143
6 1000
7 4,777,800